Food Fights

David Haslam has been a General Practitioner since
1976. He writes and broadcasts regularly on medical
topics and is a frequent contributor to *Practical
Parenting*. He is the author of six books, and is Vice
Chairman of the General Practitioner Writers Associ-
ation. He is a Patron of Crysis (alongside Jane Asher
and Claire Rayner), a judge for the Parent Friendly
Awards and a member of the Huggies Childcare
Panel, as well as being Chairman of the Examination
Board for the Royal College of General Practitioners.

Dr Haslam is married with two children and lives
in East Anglia. His special interests are music and
photography.

Dr David Haslam

Food Fights

A practical guide
for parents worried about
their children's eating habits

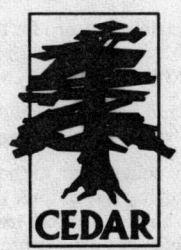

CEDAR

A Mandarin Paperback
FOOD FIGHTS

First published in Great Britain 1986
as *Eat It Up!*
by Macdonald & Co (Publishers) Ltd
This revised and updated edition published 1995
by Mandarin Paperbacks
an imprint of Reed Consumer Books Ltd
Michelin House, 81 Fulham Road, London SW3 6RB
and Auckland, Melbourne, Singapore and Toronto

A CIP catalogue record for this title
is available from the British Library
ISBN 0 7493 2065 6

Printed and bound in Great Britain
by Cox & Wyman Ltd, Reading, Berkshire

For Barbara,
Katy and Christopher

Contents

Acknowledgements

I could not have written this book without the assistance and advice of a great many people. In particular I would like to thank all those parents who wrote to me about their experiences, all the authors whose research I have quoted, and the many representatives of official organizations who took the time and trouble to let me know their views. I am particularly grateful to Tam Fry, of the Child Growth Foundation, for permission to reproduce the growth centile charts. More than anything, I am grateful to my wife, Barbara, and my two children, Katy and Christopher. I might have learnt a great deal about feeding problems and the science of nutrition from textbooks and research papers, but I learnt even more from having a family. I can't thank them enough.

Introduction

*'Every mealtime it's the same. When we do manage
to sit her at the table she looks miserably at the meal
and takes one mouthful which she chews for ages.
Eventually she spits it back on her plate. I simply
dread mealtimes now. What on earth am I doing
wrong?'*

Mother of a 3-year-old

It's all so very frustrating. You have all the right intentions, read the views of all the experts, and have made up
your mind that your child is going to eat sensibly and
healthily. You aren't going to be one of those parents
whose children eat nothing but hamburgers and chips,
with sweets between meals.

So, what happens? Your child sits at the table, refusing
to eat one mouthful of the 'good food' you've given him,
and stirs at it with a fork until its cold and inedible
anyway. He then goes out to play with his friends and
they all merrily share out the sweets that the others have
been given. When he comes in to watch TV he is
bombarded with adverts for fizzy drinks and junk food. It
makes you want to scream.

Before a child is born, everyone has their idea of what
sort of parent he or she is going to be. It's so easy to see
the mistakes that other parents are making. You aren't

going to be one of them. It's only a matter of being firm, after all. If you bring your child up correctly from the start then surely you won't have the problems these other parents have. That's the theory anyway.

Countless parents decide that their child won't eat between meals, won't eat junk food, won't have the TV on at mealtimes, and will eat fruit rather than sweets. Unfortunately, as in so many other areas of parenthood, one thing is overlooked. It's all well and good the parent deciding how things are going to be, but no one gets the child's agreement in advance. After all, if only children had to sign a contract before birth in which they would agree to eat properly, sleep through the night, and not repeat rude words in front of granny, then life would be infinitely easier.

Feeding problems are one of the major concerns of parents. Not only do they worry that their child will come to harm from refusing the food he is given, but they feel desperately upset that after all the effort they put into preparing the food, the child who won't eat is also rejecting them as well. For the young child feeding is entirely the parents' responsibility, and when things seem to be going wrong parents feel this responsibility very heavily.

Incidentally, rather than writing 'he or she' every time I mention the child in this book, I will simply write 'he'. This is only to make the book easier to read. Boys don't cause more problems. Similarly I won't write 'mother or father' each time, but just 'mother', as mothers are more often the ones doing the feeding. In no way am I implying that fathers do not have an important role to play. They do.

If you look at TV advertisements, a mother is often shown as the provider of food. She appears at the table with some dish or other, and the smiles and 'oohs' of the family show that this mum is certainly a success. Compare that with the real life scene we have all faced over and over again. The mother has worked all morning, preparing some special new meal. She brings it to the table. The kids groan, ask 'What on earth's that?', or else go 'Yuk', and – without even tasting a mouthful – say 'I don't like it. Can't we have fish fingers?'

It's no wonder that parents get upset. After all if the image of a good mother is one who succeeds at feeding, child rearing, and so on, then is it any wonder that parents who have less success – and that's pretty well everyone – decide they must be inadequate?

The problem isn't helped by friends and relatives who watch all the goings-on at the table, 'tut tut' under their breath and later tell you that you're being too soft.

While researching this book I asked readers of *Parents* magazine to contact me if they had experienced problems feeding their children. I was inundated with letters, and I will regularly quote from them throughout the book. The frustration that comes over from so many of these parents is intense. Take these few examples from a selection of the letters.

'My six-and-a-half-year-old has been a "picky eater" since starting solid feeding. The fights, the pleading, and the waste have been dreadful.'

'Our two-year-old son drove us both mad. He was always refusing to eat foods that he had eaten perfectly happily a couple of days earlier. When we said he had to eat it, he always complained of tummy ache, and frequently would be sick to prove it.'

'It would be lovely if for once my son would say "I'm hungry. What's for lunch?", but he doesn't. He's just not interested. Whatever I do, he doesn't want to eat. I could weep.'

As a parent I experienced exactly the same frustrations with our two children. My wife, Barbara, and I went through months of despairing that we would ever get them to eat properly. One of them went through a maddening phase of virtually refusing all food for a week at a time, and then following it by a week of devouring everything in sight. On other occasions we faced the frustration of having a child who would pick at a meal for ages, claiming not to be hungry, and yet five minutes later be back in the kitchen asking for a biscuit. A medical training gave me little formal instruction in how to deal with children's feeding problems, but being a parent taught my wife and me a great deal. We have all survived the trial of picky children and in this book I will be drawing on our own experiences, as well as quoting from other parents, and looking at the views of the experts.

Experts, of course, cause a lot of the confusion and worry. They just don't seem to be able to make their minds up about food. One minute something is good for you, and the next it is labelled as a potential killer.

When I was a small boy I frequently had a meal that parents in the 1950s were told was full of goodness – the perfect healthy diet. You probably had it too. It was that simple childhood meal of a boiled egg, salt, toast soldiers, and a glass of milk – preferably a good and creamy glass of 'gold top'.

So what happened? Parents nowadays constantly get bombarded with advice on diet and would realize that the egg yolk has been shown to increase the cholesterol in the blood, the salt has been linked with high blood pressure, the sliced bread – which in those days was rarely wholemeal – has been labelled as a junk food, and the butter spread on it has been linked with heart disease. As far as I know, the eggshell has not yet been blamed for anything, but the glass of milk certainly has.

Indeed there hardly seems to be a single food that someone somewhere hasn't blamed for something.

The average parent, as a result, finds him or herself being caught between the high powered advertising of the fast food companies, and the disdainful looks of the muesli and yoghurt brigade. Don't worry. I'm certainly not going to take the killjoy line that children should only ever eat wholefoods, never eat sweets, and should always munch brown rice instead of chips. Those parents that I know who do take that sort of approach never seem to be aware of just what their children eat the moment the parents are out of sight. If they did, it would give them the heart attack their 'health foods' are trying to prevent.

Instead, I hope to take a practical viewpoint, based on the latest reliable research, but tempered with common sense. After all, it's no good saying that if the experts keep changing their minds, it doesn't matter what sort of food you eat. The old cliché is true – you are what you eat. Without a shadow of a doubt, your diet *can* affect heart disease, cancer, strokes, diabetes, high blood pressure, tooth decay, and obesity.

The aim of this book is to look at almost all the feeding problems that worry parents. Research has shown that sleeping problems and feeding problems are the two most frequent topics on which advice is sought from health visitors, welfare clinics, and GPs by parents. Unfortunately studies have also suggested that some of the advice offered from these sources is not always particularly helpful to the worried mother. As in my book, *Sleepless Children*, which looked at the other most common child care problem, my aim will be to present the problems as seen by parents, rather than professionals, and the tips, advice, and comments of those who have found a solution, along with the best of the conclusions from research workers and other experts.

I do not intend to look at the diet and feeding of infants in this book. The whole question of breastfeeding versus bottle feeding, and of the beginnings of weaning, are dealt with admirably in many other child care books. Instead I am concentrating on the problems of children of toddler age and upward.

The book will initially consider the whole question of what a good diet is, and how children should grow and develop. The frustrating problem of food refusal, how different families deal with meal times, and the question of table manners, will be reviewed at length too. I will also be covering problems such as obesity, eating out, tummy aches, and food fads. The controversial topic of food allergies worries many parents and I hope to offer some guidance on this.

However, one of the most important messages from the book is a very simple one. Parents with feedings problems need not feel alone. There are an awful lot of us who know the frustration and worry that you are going through. Food should be a pleasure, but for many parents mealtimes all too often become battle times, with parents and children as the opposing forces, and the all-too-familiar war cries echoing:

'Eat it Up!'

'Shan't!'

'A Good Diet'

'It's so frustrating. He just won't eat anything except tomato soup, spaghetti, and pancakes. We've tried all sorts of other foods but he won't touch them. I'm sick with worry. What will happen to him?'

Children are quite extraordinary creatures. One day they say they love a particular food. The next day they spit it out. For weeks on end they may refuse to drink milk, and then they go to a friend's house and drink a glassful perfectly happily. It's no wonder that parents get exasperated.

Any consideration of children's feeding problems must start by taking a look at the whole question of what a 'good diet' should be. If parents have some understanding of nutrition then some of their children's fads and fancies may become much less worrying. As we will see, good nutrition can be had from the strangest choices of food, and some of the foods you may have thought essential may actually be relatively unimportant. Indeed you may have been very worried that he doesn't eat something that in fact he doesn't really need. Your child's diet may be better than you think.

Nevertheless, this book is not meant to be a highly detailed textbook of nutrition. Instead the aim of this first section is simply to summarize current views on the best foods to offer your child. Even if you find it difficult to get your child to eat a good choice of foods every day, you should be able to plan ahead so that over a week or fortnight your child will get an acceptable overall diet.

There are other reasons to have some understanding of nutrition. Whilst a young child's diet is obviously completely controlled by his parents, by school age in many families the mother often is choosing only a third of her child's meals. Breakfasts may be snatched by each member of the family individually, or even ignored completely. Indeed in 40 per cent of American families the parents have nothing to do with their children's breakfast. Lunch may be provided at school, with any choice being made by the child. It is only the evening meal where the mother may again 'take control'. Children who have absorbed some of the principles of good nutrition early in life will make better choices as they get older.

The problem with so many books and articles on diet is that they don't seem to have anything to do with the real world. Is there really any value in charts telling you how many milligrams of vitamin E a seven-year-old should eat each day, or the phosphorus requirements of a three-year-old? Such information is readily available elsewhere, but if your problem is getting your four-year-old to eat anything at all except fish fingers, then such charts are unlikely to be much use.

Believe it or not, food should be fun. The last thing any parent should do is get so worried about their child's diet that the kitchen takes on the air of a laboratory with the mother ticking off the daily requirements of vitamins, minerals, and so on, as she offers food to her children. Don't get too obsessed about it all. If you follow the few basic principles, and if your child is happy, healthy, and growing, it is most unlikely that his diet is terribly wrong.

There are of course parents and nutritionists who would

disagree with me. 'Your child may look healthy,' they sometimes say, 'but how do you know he wouldn't be even better if only you gave him this or that vitamin supplement.' I consider that to be a completely unjustified argument. It saddens me to see the vast amount of unnecessary vitamin supplements, and the like, that are advertised and sold with no real evidence of their value. There are, of course, occasions when such obsessional attention to diet is important – diseases such as coeliac disease or cystic fibrosis are examples – but for the vast majority of children an excellent diet can be obtained from ordinary everyday foods.

One common worry about trying to offer your family a 'good diet' is that it will be expensive. Parents frequently say to me that they know what their children should be eating but 'how can we afford good foods like beef on our income?' I am happy to say that there is no need for concern, and in fact a good diet may well turn out to be cheaper than a poor one. In general fresh foods are better than convenience foods and they are usually cheaper. Unfortunately fresh foods are rarely advertised, but it is advertising that often pushes up the price of the packaged foods. Parents may spend a large proportion of their money on meat to provide protein, but because of their low income they buy cheap cuts of meat. They are making the mistake of thinking that meat is essential. The cheaper meats often contain mostly fat anyway, which makes them a relatively poor source of protein. The parent would be a lot better off buying cheaper non-meat protein foods.

Before dealing in detail with the various types of food, it is worth briefly considering current views on diet as a whole. Many people are confused by the constantly changing advice. However in recent years a vast amount of research has been carried out on diet and it *is* now possible to give simple and sensible guidelines. These are based on two major reports in the UK, which are themselves based on a thorough analysis of countless other world-wide reports. In September 1983, NACNE (the National Advisory Committee on Nutrition Education) produced its important 'Proposals for nutritional guidelines for health education in Britain', and in July 1984, COMA (the Committee on Medical Aspects of Food Policy) produced theirs. Their conclusions were very similar to other major reviews of diet published in the USA – in particular reports from the National Heart, Lung and Blood Institute and the American Heart Association.

Indeed, in 1994, the United States Department of Agriculture announced that American schoolchildren were eating too much fat and sodium, and too little fibre, and proposed new rules for the content of school lunches. The federal government in the USA spends more than $5bn a year to provide lunches for 25 million children in about 92,000 schools, and when the programme first began after the Second World War the chief concern was malnutrition. The focus was then on energy. It has now switched to the problem of over-consumption of fatty foods and sodium. This change in priority is typical of modern nutritional advice in most of the Western world, and is an important message of this book.

This renewed interest in the quality, rather than the quantity of food stems from the realization that diet is linked with many chronic diseases. Societies that eat similar diets tend to have similar patterns of disease, and when someone moves from one culture to another they often develop the diseases of their new homeland. The classic example is that of the Japanese who traditionally eat a relatively low-fat diet, and have a correspondingly low incidence of heart disease.

When they move to a Western culture, such as the USA, or else adopt a more Western, meat-eating lifestyle

4

at home in Japan, their chance of developing heart disease increases. The particular form of heart trouble most closely connected with diet is arteriosclerosis – the narrowing of arteries due to layers of cholesterol being laid down in a similar fashion to the furring up of water pipes. The fact that this is something that develops throughout one's lifetime, rather than coming on suddenly, was shown horrifyingly in the Korean War. The average age of the American soldiers killed in the war was only twenty-two. Of these, thirty-five per cent already had significant arteriosclerosis of the coronary arteries – the vital arteries that feed the heart.

Faced with evidence like this, and more and more research that changing one's diet can lessen many of these problems, most Western families do need to rethink their diets and follow the sort of advice laid down in the NACNE or COMA reports. Ill health isn't usually due to chance. Bodies need looking after all their lives. It's no good waiting till diseases have happened to do something about their causes.

So – what is the advice that is going to make such a difference to all our lives? Is it complicated and expensive? Will the kids eat it, anyway?

Incredibly it couldn't really be simpler. The rules are these:

Eat less fat, sugar, and salt.
Eat more fibre.

That is it. Nothing more and nothing less. There are no lists of essential vitamins, minerals, and different sorts of proteins that everyone must eat. Indeed the whole concept of the 'balanced diet' was virtually abandoned in the NACNE report, and for very good reasons.

The traditional teaching on what families should eat was based on the theory that, without advice, many

5

children and adults would not get enough of certain vital foods. That certainly used to be true, and it remains true for people on very low incomes, some adults on very faddy diets, and some elderly people who live alone. However, for the huge majority of families in the affluent West, problems rarely arise from a lack of nutrients. Instead diets tend to be unbalanced because there is too much, not too little, of a particular foodstuff.

Few people now need to worry about their children not getting enough Vitamin A, but tens of thousands ought to worry about their getting too much sugar.

Most of the books on child care that I have ever looked at have carried worrying-looking lists of the diseases that result from living on diets which lack some of the minerals, vitamins, and trace elements, along with lists of foods that can provide good sources of these. Don't worry, I'm not going to worry or bore you with charts like that here. The vast majority of children – even when going through their faddy phases – still get enough of the essential foodstuffs. Certainly if you look at an individual day then many children will not get their average daily requirements of many nutrients. But – and this point is essential – taken over a period of time, and to many people's surprise, what a child eats and what he needs are actually remarkably similar.

This is one of the essential rules of feeding. Don't take too narrow a view. Don't worry about your child's eating as judged by just a day or a week. Take a broad viewpoint. Similarly, if you are hoping to follow the new dietary guidelines then don't panic if your child wants an iced bun or a chocolate bar. An occasional 'treat' like that will do no harm. A chocolate bar every day for months on end quite possibly will. Average intakes count, not individual meals or days. You will see how important this is when I consider 'food fads' in more detail later.

6

Traditionally foods have been divided into three main groups – carbohydrate, protein, and fat. Protein has been described as good for growth and repair of the body. Carbohydrates are said to be energy-giving, and fats to be essential for providing certain vitamins – as well as being important in making food more palatable and in helping the body remain healthy. For many people, descriptions like this are the sum total of their knowledge of nutrition – through no fault of their own. Countless articles on diet – or, more usually, on dieting – reinforce these ideas.

These subdivisions are frequently useless. Take cheese, for example. Everyone knows, thanks to advertising, that a good piece of cheese is a splendid source of protein. In fact it may also be an even better source of fat. Fats themselves have a remarkably high energy value – more than twice as many calories as sugar or flour. It's confusing, isn't it?

Indeed, the NACNE report suggested that it was time to discard these different food groups, describing them as 'of little relevance to current nutritional thinking'.

What is vitally important is for your child to have a varied diet. As I have already mentioned, if your child misses a particular nutrient at one meal or another, the chances are that he will make up for it later. If he does eat food of a reasonable variety over a period of time, and – this is most important – if he is growing normally, then it is incredibly unlikely that he is missing out on some important foodstuff. In Chapter 4 I will look at some of the few exceptions, but must stress that these are extremely rare.

All this is, of course, very good news to the worried parent. You can throw out all those charts of daily requirements and lists of the best sources of riboflavin or panthothenic acid. They've never made sense to me,

7

anyway. If you know for example how much protein is in half a pound of bacon, does that mean lean, or streaky, and if lean – how lean? Does it make any difference how you cook it? Do you have to take into account the scraps left on the plate? Of course you don't – or at least, you can't.

This whole idea may even seem too revolutionary for you. Can we really trust our children to get reasonable nutrition if we just rely on them to eat a variety of foods? To show that you can I will return to the traditional major subdivisions of food, protein, fat, and carbohydrate. I will deal with calcium, as an example of the many important minerals in the diet, and also consider the calories in our food. In the next chapter I will be looking at vitamins, but let us now review the other groups one at a time.

Protein

For a child who is offered as much food as he wants a shortage of protein is really remarkably rare. That is because of the wide variety of foods that contain protein.

You may have heard of first- and second-class proteins. To my mind these descriptions are valuable for scientists, but a hindrance for parents. All proteins are made up of amino-acids. Some of these proteins cannot be made by the body but must be eaten ready-made. Fish, meat, milk and dairy products all provide these 'first-class proteins'. However, other foods contain amino-acids which the body can then combine together to make into protein – the badly termed 'second-class protein'. There is nothing second-class about them at all. The proteins provided in this way by nuts, beans, bread, or potatoes can be just as valuable as the 'first-class' ones.

8

So, even if your child refuses to eat meat from the butcher's – as many children do – he may well eat a hot dog sausage (which contains animal protein), in a bread roll (which contains vegetable protein).

A child who eats cake will get the protein from the egg that was used to make it. Hamburgers, fish fingers, sausages, puddings, or anything with milk in – all these contain protein. They may not be prime roast beef, but they are protein all the same.

Fats

You certainly need not worry that your child lacks fat in his diet. It is more than likely that he gets too much, as I will discuss later. Such snacks as biscuits contain fats, as do most of the 'junk foods', virtually all meats, dairy produce, pies, and so on. The body's actual requirement for fats is very small, and almost any childhood diet will supply enough. Incidentally, fats do make you feel full when you've eaten them. Chinese food is low in fat – which is why you so often feel hungry again half an hour after a Chinese meal!

Carbohydrates

There are three main types of carbohydrate – sugars, starches, and the undigestible form found in dietary fibre. There is certainly no likelihood that any child has a diet deficient in carbohydrate. You only have to consider the number of products that contain sugar to realize just how much carbohydrate your child eats. Look at the ingredients listed on the tins and packets in your kitchen cupboard. Sugar will appear in a huge number of them including tomato ketchup, baked beans, and tinned vegetables.

While very few children fail to eat enough carbohydrate, very many eat too much of the wrong sorts and a brief look at carbohydrates in more detail is worthwhile.

All sugars and starches have the same basic constituents. The sugars are made up of single molecules – the monosaccharides glucose, fructose, and galactose – or double molecules, the disaccharides. The disaccharides are combinations of the monosaccharides. For instance lactose is a combination of glucose and galactose, and sucrose is a combination of glucose and fructose.

The starches are more complicated, consisting of branched chains of large numbers of glucose molecules. However the body eventually breaks all the carbohydrates back down to their constituents.

As well as subdividing the carbohydrates like this, you can also consider them as 'refined' – sometimes known as 'processed' – or 'natural'. As their name implies, the natural carbohydrates come ready provided by nature and are always combined in foods that also give other important nutrients. Refined carbohydrates are often just added to other foods and provide nothing except calories. There is absolutely no doubt that almost everyone eats too many refined sugars, and not enough natural carbohydrate in the form of sugars and starches. I will be looking again at sugar consumption later in this chapter, but my aim in this first section has been to show that parents need not fear that their children will not get enough carbohydrates. They will. If the proportion of carbohydrate taken as starches is increased, your children will benefit all the more. If you offer your child more bread, potatoes, pasta, and vegetables and less sugar, sweets, biscuits, and cake you will be going a long way towards improving the quality of the carbohydrate in his diet.

Calories

Calories are simply a measure of the energy value of food. The more Calories a given food contains, the more energy it provides for the body. Most people are very familiar with this idea, as Calorie control is a favourite way of slimming. If you eat more Calories than your body uses up in energy, you get fat – and vice versa.

As Calories are units of measurement that most people understand, I am listing the average daily requirements of Calories at different ages in Table I. It must be realized

Table I Recommended Daily Calorie Requirements

Boys and Girls	0–1 year	800
	1–2 years	1200
	2–3 years	1400
	3–5 years	1600
	5–7 years	1800
	7–9 years	2100
Boys	9–12 years	2500
	12–15 years	2800
	15–18 years	3000
Girls	9–12 years	2300
	12–15 years	2300
	15–18 years	2300
Men	18–35 years depending on activity	2700–3600
Women	18–55 years (most occupations)	2200
	pregnancy (second half)	2400
	breast feeding	2700

that these *are* only averages, based on recommendations by the Department of Health and Social Security in the UK and similar recommendations in the USA. There is a wide range, depending on size and activity levels. They are, however, of interest as a guideline.

If your child is well, and is growing normally, then he must be getting enough Calories. As one mother wrote to me: 'I really can't understand it. Emma [her three-year-old daughter] hardly seems to eat a thing. She just picks at her food, nibbles a bit when the fancy takes her, but never has a proper meal. Despite that, the doctor says she is growing perfectly. She certainly looks all right.'

Countless parents will echo this worry, and yet Emma *must be* getting enough Calories from somewhere. Bodies don't grow without food. Many parents don't realize quite how highly Calories can be concentrated. For example one french fried potato contains as many Calories as two or three boiled potatoes. The fat adds the Calories – foods with a lot of fat in have the highest concentration of Calories. This is certainly not always a good thing, but I am here only showing that parents rarely need worry that their child is undernourished.

Calcium

As everyone knows, calcium is essential for strong teeth and bones. It is only one of the many minerals that the body needs, but probably the most important. Of the calcium in your body, about 98 per cent is in the bones, one per cent in the teeth, and the rest in the muscles and blood.

As well as being present in cheese, citrus fruits, cereals,

bread, and some vegetables, by far the best source of calcium is milk. A pint a day provides all the calcium (not to mention protein) that your child needs.

I can hear the moans already. 'A pint a day! My child won't touch the stuff. I just can't make him drink it.' It is an understandable worry – until you consider the foods in which he may be actually taking milk without noticing. There are scrambled eggs, rice puddings, pancakes, mashed or creamed potatoes, omelettes, ice-cream, custard, and all the other milky puddings – not to mention the milk he may have on cereal. With a selection of foods like that it is again very unlikely that your child is lacking calcium in his diet. The other minerals are equally unlikely to be missing.

The whole question of vitamins, and the need for supplements, confuses and worries many parents and I will deal with these separately in the next chapter. However as for all the other important constituents of food, you should now realize that if your child is growing satisfactorily – something you can check up on in Chapter 3 – then he is almost certainly getting enough. Instead of listing things that your child must eat, attention nowadays has switched to the new dietary guidelines that I mentioned earlier – less fat, less sugar, less salt and more fibre.

Why are these suggestions so important, and what can parents do about them? Let's look at them one at a time, and remember that this advice is directed at the whole family.

Eat less fat

More people in the Western world die from coronary artery disease than anything else. Many of them die relatively young. In 1980 a third of deaths from heart disease in England and Wales occurred in men before retirement age. Yet it is largely preventable.

Your risk, or your children's eventual risk, of suffering heart disease is controlled by several factors. You can help yourself by eating less fat, especially saturated fat, not smoking, and taking more exercise. The incidence of heart disease in the USA has recently fallen dramatically as a result of putting these simple measures into practice.

While coronary artery disease is obviously rare in childhood, this does not mean that diet only becomes important later in life. Heart disease may appear 'out of the blue' to strike down a seemingly healthy middle aged man, but the seeds for such an event are sown in childhood. Incidentally, please don't feel that this means it is too late for *you* to change your diet, even if you change your children's. It's never too late and there is increasing evidence that early damage can be slowly undone.

Certain families are particularly predisposed to coronary artery disease, people with far too much cholesterol in their blood. Doctors can check for this simply by a blood test, but the dietary advice given to such families applies equally to everyone else. A few people do need very strict diets indeed, even occasionally with drug treatment to reduce their blood cholesterol, but though it was once thought that everyone else could eat what fat they wanted, we now know that reducing fat in the diet helps everyone prevent heart disease. The particularly dangerous type of fat is saturated fat, and eating too much of this increases the amount of cholesterol in the blood. The more cholesterol in the blood, the greater the risk of heart disease.

Saturated fats are mainly found in red meats, dairy products and most margarines; polyunsaturated fats are mainly found in vegetable oils. The fat in poultry is much less saturated than other animal fats. (Incidentally, the more saturated the fat is, the harder it is at room temperature.)

Cholesterol is also present in the diet, particularly in egg yolks, and to a lesser extent meat and dairy foods. There is no cholesterol in plant foods. However, cutting down on the amount of cholesterol you eat in the form of eggs is far less important than cutting down on saturated fats generally. Increasingly evidence is accumulating that physical exercise does help control the harmful effects of some types of fat.

Of course, many people are already aware that 'fat is bad for them' and have reduced the amount in their family's diet. However, there is far more in our food than meets the eye. In whole (silver top) milk, 52 per cent of the calories are made up of fat. Full fat yogurt is the same. Butter is 100 per cent fat. Bacon is 60–80 per cent depending on whether you trim off the fat or not, and Cheddar cheese is 71 per cent. Sausages are about 70 per cent fat.

However you needn't panic. No one is suggesting you abandon all these foods. It's a question of balance: follow these simple tips and you will successfully reduce the amount of fat in your family's diet.

- Grill, don't fry.
- Cut the visible fat off meat before you cook it.
- Reduce the amount of full fat cheese, butter and cream you eat.
- Change from full cream milk to fresh skimmed milk. (Though for under-fives, see the advice in the next section.)
- Eat less red meat, and more fish and poultry.

To return briefly to milk, more and more families are

switching to skimmed milk from whole fat milk. Skimmed milk sales in Britain rose by 38 per cent in 1984, and as a pint of whole milk contains 22.2 gm of fat and a pint of skimmed milk contains 0.6 gm of fat this can only be a good thing. However, many people find the taste of skimmed milk too watery, and for them semi-skimmed milk, with a fat content of 9.1 gm per pint, is a very worthwhile compromise. It has plenty of flavour and is well worth trying even if you have already sampled one bottle of skimmed milk and thrown it out in disgust! Who knows, you may eventually find the transition from semi-skimmed to skimmed relatively painless.

Table 2 The Breakdown of the Three Commonest Types of Milk

	Fat g	Energy Calories	Protein g	Calcium Mg	Vitamin B_2 Mg	Vitamin A Micro-grams	Vitamin D Micro-grams
Whole Milk	22.2	380	19.3	702	1.11	228	0.13
Semi-skimmed Milk	9.1	266	19.6	725	1.13	89	0.05
Skimmed Milk	0.6	193	19.9	761	1.17	Trace	Trace

A brief warning. Skimmed milk is definitely not suitable for infants, who need the high energy content of the fuller fat milks. Children up to the age of four or five are probably better with some full fat milk, or even semi-skimmed milk, to provide vitamins A and D (see Chapter 3), though obviously this depends on what other vitamins they have. Indeed some low fat milks have added vitamins, though these are all sold under trade names. In addition, for a very young child to get enough calories from skimmed milk, the amount of milk that needs to be drunk will result in an unacceptable increase in sodium intake.

If your family is going to eat less fat they obviously must get their energy from somewhere. The answer is to eat more potatoes, pasta, rice, vegetables, and fruit in the diet. Which conveniently brings me to the next important bit of advice

Eat more fibre

Too little fibre (we used to call it 'roughage') in the diet has been linked to a whole host of diseases – amongst them appendicitis, constipation, diverticular disease, piles, varicose veins, and even possibly some forms of bowel cancer.

Please don't increase your family's fibre intake by buying fibre tablets, or other expensive supplements. It is far easier to get your family eating more fresh fruit and vegetables, more potatoes and other root crops, and more peas and beans. Eat more bread – so long as it is high in fibre. Wholemeal is best, but if your children are as 'addicted' to sliced white bread as most then you can start by using white bread with added fibre – there are several on the market. My children still embarrassingly seem to think of white bread as being a special treat, but will eat a really good wholemeal loaf enthusiastically. The secret lies in finding a really tasty one – or even baking your own. There are some pretty tasteless chewy loaves on the market that children are wise to refuse, but don't just try one sort of wholemeal loaf and give up if they won't eat it.

Wholemeal breakfast cereals and muesli can also be good sources of fibre – although some commercial mueslis contain a lot of added sugar. The ingredients listed on the side of cereal packets are given in their order of quantity.

Avoid those in which sugar is given near the top of the list, however much their advertising image stresses wholesome natural goodness!

One word of caution – if you try and give children of toddler age too much fibre they will feel full very quickly and unable to eat enough of other more nourishing foods. Take it gently and ease back on the fibre foods temporarily if this seems to be happening.

Eat less sugar

Most people are at least vaguely aware that too much sugar is bad for them. However we still eat about 40 kg of sugar each every year. That is worth 150,000 Calories a year or 410 Calories a day each.

You may already have hidden the sugar bowl, and encouraged your family to avoid putting sugar on cereals and in drinks. However, the depressing news is that you are almost certainly still eating a huge amount of sugar concealed in other foods.

The percentage of Calories that are sugar in baked beans is 31 per cent, in Coca-Cola 100 per cent, in All Bran 22 per cent, in ice-cream 55 per cent, and in tomato ketchup 94 per cent. Am I depressing you? Well, there is worse to come. Many foods contain so much saturated fat that they are only made palatable by adding sugar. Cream of tomato soup has 89 per cent of its energy supplied by fats and sugars, which makes it about as genuinely nourishing as a packet of sweets.

Cutting back on sugar will remain difficult for as long as food labels are as inadequate as they are, and only legislation will change this. However, you can control the amount of added sugar your children eat, and have fewer puddings and more fresh fruit. Choose plain biscuits and fewer sticky buns. It may take you some time as a family to lose your sweet tooth – it took me three months to enjoy a cup of coffee when I first gave up – but it's well worth it.

Eat less salt

There is plenty of evidence that too much salt is one of the causes of high blood pressure – which in itself may eventually lead to strokes and heart failure. The amount of salt we actually need is tiny, so cutting back can do no harm. As most of us get around a third of our salt from that added in cooking or at the table, then hiding the salt cellar may be all you need to do. Again, you will do your children a favour if they get used to food without lashings of salt.

Other foods with a high salt content obviously include salted peanuts and crisps, but sauces, tinned vegetables and tinned soups are also fairly high in salt, though tinned vegetables with no added salt are now on the market.

Don't try and change your family's diet too suddenly or you won't succeed. Take it gently. If you think the advice has all been a bit negative, it isn't. For everything I've suggested you have less of, there is another food that you should try and eat more. Eat less fatty meat, and more lean. Eat fewer manufactured and packaged foods, and more fruit and vegetables, pulses, pasta and good bread. Cut down on sugar and salt, and let your family discover the real taste of food again – with herbs and spices as needed.

Is it worth it? You cannot possibly give your children a better gift than a healthy start in life. What is more, it will help you and your husband or wife stay fit and healthy for far longer – and your children will be grateful for that too.

2

Vitamins and Fluoride

'My health visitor told me to give him vitamin drops every day. My doctor told me there was no need. Some of my friends give them, but most can't be bothered. It's all rather confusing. Who is right?'

Parents have an impossible task. It seems that no one can agree on the rights and wrongs of many aspects of child rearing, and as a result all manner of conflicting advice gets offered. One of the items of greatest confusion in the realm of diet is the use of vitamin and fluoride supplements. I've coupled these together in the same chapter not because they are similar chemicals which they aren't – but because drops and tablets of both are widely available, and parents need to know when and how to use them.

Vitamins are essential. The body cannot function efficiently without them, and if they are missing from the diet their lack can cause a number of very serious illnesses. Luckily they are only required in tiny amounts each day, measured in thousandths of a gram or much less. Indeed the total amount of vitamins an adult requires adds up to about an eighth of a teaspoonful each day.

Vitamins are also big business. Certain people have developed the idea that if a tiny amount of a vitamin does you good, then taking more must be even better. Many men and women take large doses in the hope that the extra vitamins will both prevent them becoming ill, and make them even healthier. It would be marvellous if it were true, but there is little evidence that such megadoses help, and a lot of evidence that they can be harmful.

Not only can you buy vast numbers of different vitamin supplements from chemists and 'health food' shops but you can also buy books which explain how you can treat many childhood problems by giving vitamins. One such guide advises vitamin E for warts, vitamin B for dandruff, and vitamin D for conjunctivitis. As these are all conditions that frequently recover with no treatment whatsoever then I am not surprised that people who recommend such treatments claim good results.

Such ideas are generally not endorsed by the vast majority of paediatricians and nutritionists. While there can be no guarantee that they are right, nevertheless my reading of the subject leads me to agree with one of Britain's most respected paediatricians, Dr Hugh Jolly, who said 'in the case of vitamins more is not better – it is useless and can even be harmful.'

There are many important vitamins, and I will deal with them one by one. I do not intend to look at the more controversial so-called vitamins that some writers mention – such as vitamin T and vitamin U – as so little is genuinely known about them and they are certainly not essential to our diet.

The main vitamins are divided into two groups: the water-soluble, and the fat-soluble. The various forms of vitamin B, as well as vitamin C, can be dissolved in water, while vitamins A, D, E and K are soluble in fats and oils. The importance of this distinction is that A, D, E and K can be stored in the body dissolved in our fat, but the others are not. The water-soluble vitamins are also likely to be lost in food preparation, and cooking. A great deal of vitamin C may be washed down the drain with the cooking water, instead of making its way into your family's bodies.

As fat-soluble vitamins can be stored in the body fat, they can build up to toxic levels if too much is consumed – a danger that may increase if people continue to take megadoses of vitamin supplements. Mind you, vitamin supplements are by no means new. Many of today's parents were regularly given their spoonful of cod liver oil, or dose of Virol or Haliborange when they were children.

The most important vitamins for parents to consider are vitamins A, B, C and D.

Vitamin A

Vitamin A helps to keep the lining of the urinary tract, the lungs, and the bowel healthy, and as a result is able to help the body resist infection. However there is no evidence that extra vitamin A will prevent more infections. It can't and won't. As everyone knows, it also has a connection with eyesight. A deficiency of vitamin A can lead to night blindness, but eating extra vitamin A does not help you see better in the dark. I'm afraid another old story must bite the dust!

It is present in milk, butter, cheese and fortified margarines although the best source is liver. Carrots contain a chemical called carotene from which the body can make its own vitamin A. Eggs, tomatoes and dark green vegetables can also be a useful source.

Cod liver oil is a very concentrated way of giving vitamin A, but please do not exceed the recommended dose. Too much of this vitamin can cause blurred vision, rashes, headaches, nausea, hair loss, and insomnia, to name just a few symptoms! Don't worry though, it is virtually impossible to get too much vitamin A from normal foods.

Vitamin D

This vitamin is found in fish, margarine, eggs, dairy foods, and liver. However, our bodies can also make their own vitamin D when sunlight falls on the skin. If you live in a warm, sunny place where you don't need to wear many clothes then dietary vitamin D is much less important than for those who live in colder, cloudier climates.

Most white European and American children on a reasonably varied diet can make enough vitamin D in their skin to complete their needs and seldom need a supplement. However dark skinned children, from Asian or African backgrounds for example, are unlikely to be able to make enough vitamin D in a climate like Britain's, and almost certainly will need supplements. I will return to the whole question of supplements shortly.

Vitamin D is needed by the body to help it absorb calcium and phosphorous from the diet. These are obviously important for strong bones and teeth, and growing children understandably need a lot of it – far more than adults. Insufficient vitamin D can cause rickets, or softening of the bones and teeth. If the child walks on soft bones they bow outwards. Such bow legs used to be a common sight, but thankfully are much less of a problem nowadays although they still occur in inner cities, especially among Asian children.

Vitamin B

There are many different B vitamins. These are B$_1$ (Thiamine), B$_2$ (Riboflavin), B$_3$ (Niacin or Nicotinic Acid), B$_6$ (Pyridoxine), and B$_{12}$ (Cobalamin). You probably recognize some of the names from the sides of cereal packets. As they tend to occur together in similar foods I don't intend to deal with them each separately.

The foods that they are most commonly found in are dairy produce, yeast (and therefore spreads like Marmite), liver, potatoes, pork and other meats, wholemeal bread, eggs, and cereals. The B vitamins are essential for growth and general good health, and supplements are useful for treating many disorders in adults. However children only very rarely have a deficiency of any of the B vitamins in their diet in developed countries, although a fussy toddler on a very faddy diet might just possibly need supplements.

Vitamin C

Vitamin C helps the body fight infections, but despite numerous claims megadoses have not been proved to help prevent infections, such as colds. As everyone knows, it is mainly found in fruit and vegetables. The best sources are citrus fruits such as oranges, lemons, and grapefruit. However, potatoes also contain vitamin C, as do tomatoes and green vegetables.

There is virtually no vitamin C in cereals, squash, dairy products, fish, cheese, and eggs, so it is certainly possible for faddy children not to get enough. However, don't forget that potatoes, especially if left in their skins, do provide this vitamin so even non-fruit eaters won't go completely short. Frozen fruit and vegetables contain as much vitamin C as fresh foods, and possibly even more as they are frozen soon after they are picked, whereas the fresh may take a long time to reach the table and the vitamin C may have deteriorated.

Remembering that vitamin C is soluble in water; use as little water as possible for cooking vegetables and you will lose less.

Finally, if your children won't eat fresh fruit, don't forget fruit drinks. Many contain added vitamin C. In addition, the popularity of pure unsweetened orange juice, usually sold in cartons, has increased immensely in recent years. Parents often wonder if such juices – which are heat-treated to give them a long shelf life – contain a significant amount of vitamin C. The US citrus industry investigated this when they examined 2500 fresh oranges and found the vitamin C content to vary from 26 to 84 mg per 100 ml of juice. The average content was 55 mg per 100 ml. By contrast, the orange juices sold in long-life cartons contain 37 mg of vitamin C per 100 ml. The recommended daily requirement for adults is around 30 mg., and for children from one to eight years it is 20 mg.

Heat treatment does therefore reduce the amount of vitamin C in fresh fruit juice. The actual treatment process involves the oranges being squeezed shortly after picking, the juice then being heat-treated to produce the concentrate which is frozen for shipment to the country where it will be sold. On arrival the juice is thawed out, reconstituted, and then pasteurized before filling into sterile cartons. In a way, it seems remarkable that so much vitamin C does survive this process. While freshly squeezed juice – or eating the whole fruit – is clearly ideal, the commercial juices do contain a very significant amount of the vitamin and parents can feel reassured if their children do drink such juices.

Recent research has also shown that fruit, and probably particularly vitamin C, has a very powerful effect in helping the lungs to work efficiently. The study, in adults, shows that failure to eat fresh fruit and vegetables on a regular basis reduces lung capacity to the same extent as smoking twenty cigarettes per day. It appears that both smokers and non-smokers who do not eat fresh fruit or vegetables, or else drink fruit juice at least once a week, exhale air much less quickly than those who do. It even seems likely that frequent consumption of fresh fruit and vegetables may help to protect against emphysema.

Insufficient vitamin C can cause scurvy, which is certainly very rare these days. However the *British Medical Journal* in 1983 reported a case in a twenty-four-year-old unemployed engineer who confounded his doctors with his symptoms of spontaneous bruising, loss of appetite, night sweats, and nausea. The diagnosis was made when it turned out that he had lived on peanut butter sandwiches, a little meat, and occasional chips for three years. He ate no green vegetables, had last eaten fruit four years previously, and could not remember ever having eaten an orange. It may reassure you to know that food fads rarely last quite that long! He recovered rapidly when given vitamin C.

The two other vitamins, E and K, rarely cause problems for children. Vitamin E is found in a wide variety of foods and supplements are not required for children (apart from premature babies, who can get enough from breast milk). Vitamin K is normally made by bacteria in the intestine and is needed for efficient blood clotting. These bacteria can be killed when your child takes antibiotics, although this rarely causes problems as they soon develop again, a process which can be encouraged by giving natural live yogurt.

Vitamin Supplements

Few areas of nutrition cause so many arguments. The advice given to parents can therefore be very conflicting, and I frequently found that where doctors and health visitors work together in a team one would be advising supplements while the other was not. The teaching given to student health visitors also varies from time to time and place to place.

Babies cause few disagreements. Breast milk contains enough vitamin A, B, C and D for them! Ordinary cows' milk does not have enough C and D, but commercial dried baby milks contain added vitamins. If these milks are used then no supplements are needed for the first six months, but if ordinary milk is given – as it frequently is by Asian mothers, among others – then vitamin supplements are needed. Concentrated drops containing vitamins A, C and D are probably the easiest way to give these but the dose must not be exceeded. Fish liver oils can also be useful.

For older infants and children the advice is less clear-cut. In practice most mothers stop giving vitamin supplements once their child is eating a reasonably mixed diet. A child who takes a pint of milk a day, in drinks and other foods, and who eats fresh fruit, vegetables, or fruit juices does not need supplements. If you start to give strained foods and other solids much before six months, your child will probably be taking less milk as a result and vitamin supplements are probably useful at this change-over time.

With the older child who may be going through a 'faddy eating' stage, you may be worried that he is not getting enough vitamins. If, having read the first part of this chapter, he seems to be getting a reasonable variety of the

27

vitamin-containing foods, then there is almost certainly no need for supplements. If you are in doubt, then give a daily supplement. It is much easier than either doing immensely complicated calculations to work out if he's getting enough, or else fretting that he will come to harm. If you are worried about his diet, he will be less relaxed about meal times and faddyness may well worsen and continue for longer. The vitamin drops are an easy way of being certain he gets enough and – provided you stick to the right amount – are harmless.

Asian children, who are living away from a climate where enough natural sunlight falls on their skin to make vitamin D, certainly need vitamin supplements. In addition many Asian families use ordinary, rather than fortified, milk and social and religious customs often prevent much exposure to what sunlight there is. As well as Asians, families on very strict vegetarian diets (which can include Rastafarians) and children on prolonged treatment with the anticonvulsants Phenytoin or Phenobarbitone, will probably need vitamin D supplements.

In recent years, a great many other claims have been made for vitamin supplements. In particular, in 1988, a BBC television programme reported a study which appeared to show an increase in non-verbal IQ scores in children taking a particular vitamin supplement. This programme, and much subsequent enthusiasm and marketing, was based on a paper published in the medical journal, *The Lancet*. However within a few weeks, large numbers of nutritionists, statisticians, and other scientists had thrown very grave doubts on the findings. At the end of all the controversy there seemed to be no doubt that special vitamin supplements are of no value at all in boosting a child's intelligence. This was confirmed by a further study of vitamin and mineral supplementation in eighty-six children aged 11–13 and published in 1990. The conclusion was clear: 'Vitamin and mineral supplementation does not improve the performance of school-children in tests of reasoning'. By all means ensure that your child has a good diet, but don't waste your money on pills and potions.

In summary, I would recommend supplements for babies who are weaned much earlier than six months, for Asian children in Western societies, and for children whose parents are worried about their eating habits. For these last the vitamins may not be essential, but the parental worry itself may cause problems, and supplements are an easy way of solving them. A reasonably mixed diet will give your child enough vitamins. A mixed diet and a supplement will not overdose him, but extra supplements above recommended dose levels may do more harm than good.

Fluoride

As with the vitamins, there is argument and controversy as to whether the use of fluoride supplements is necessary and helpful. Most people are now well aware that fluoride can do a great deal to strengthen the enamel of your child's teeth and help the teeth to resist the acids that cause tooth decay.

Tooth decay, or caries, is a very preventable disease. It is certainly not something that will happen inevitably to your or your children's teeth. To a large extent it is caused by bacteria which are invariably present in the mouth and can form a sticky gluey substance on the teeth, called plaque. The plaque then absorbs sugar from foods like sweets, and the bacteria turn the sugar into acid. This acid begins to corrode the teeth.

Obviously the less sugar that there is in your child's diet, the less acid will be made by these bacteria. Equally obviously, the less plaque there is, the less can any acid be produced. Regular cleaning of teeth, use of dental floss, and disclosing tablets to reveal the hidden plaque will be of tremendous value. However, you and I are living in the real world. It is tremendously difficult for children to clean their teeth after every meal – particularly after school meals. However much you may discourage sweets, sweets will be handed round by friends, and short of moving to a desert island you will be hard pressed to ban them altogether.

However, all is not lost as an adequate supply of fluoride in your child's diet may give a great deal of protection against caries. This very definitely does not mean that diet and tooth cleaning can be ignored, but it certainly does help. Many people live in areas where there is sufficient natural fluoride in the drinking water. The best way of checking up on this is to contact your local Water or Health Authorities, or by contacting the Community Dental Service. Your doctor or dentist will almost certainly have the information too. You cannot rely on anyone to tell you without your asking, however.

If your questions reveal that there is insufficient fluoride in your drinking water, then you need to think about supplements. A level of around one part of fluoride to a million parts of water will certainly mean you do not need them.

Fluoride supplements are available in several different forms – particularly tablets, drops, or mouth washes. Some dentists will apply topical applications of fluoride containing varnishes twice a year. It is essential that you do not give supplements to your child without checking first that he needs them. Too much fluoride can lead to an unsightly mottling of the teeth (fluorosis). Obviously it is essential not to exceed the recommended dosage.

Here lies a considerable problem. Ninety-eight per cent

of toothpaste available today contains fluoride. There is concern that if children swallow the toothpaste in addition to taking fluoride tablets or drops then fluorosis might result. The simplest answer to this dilemma would be to give a supplement when the water levels justify it, and to use a non-fluoride toothpaste. Such pastes are however frequently unobtainable. Perhaps the best solution is to find a dentist with an interest in preventive dentistry for children and discuss your particular problem with him or her. He or she will know the local circumstances best. Incidentally, if the water in your area does contain enough fluoride, then fluoride-containing pastes are still perfectly safe. The risk of fluorosis from swallowing toothpaste is tiny.

What do dentists do for their own children? An interesting study in London in 1981 showed that sugar consumption had been successfully restricted in 81 per cent of their families and 84 per cent of these children had caries-free teeth at age eleven or older. The study concluded that sugar restriction was regarded by the dentists as far more important than fissure sealing, fluoride applications, or fluoride tablets. As in Chapter 1, the 'eat less sugar' message seems to be coming over loud and clear. At present in the United Kingdom the average person consumes approximately 40 kg of sugar each year – almost 2 lb each week. However, times are changing. In Switzerland – a country which produces some of the world's best chocolate – the Swiss Office of Health allows certain confectionery products to be advertised as 'safe for teeth' provided they do not cause tooth-dissolving acids. Such labelling would certainly be an advantage elsewhere too.

3

Normal Growth

'I weigh Matthew every week, and get dreadfully worried about his progress. Some weeks he puts some weight on, but on others he stays still or even loses. Is there anything I can do to keep him growing steadily?'

It is not surprising that parents get concerned about their children's growth. It is one of the few ways in which they can see that their love, care, and attention is doing some good. 'My, how he's grown,' is a remarkably common comment by friends and relations who have not seen your child for a while, while occasional queries – frequently from grandparents – of 'Are you sure you're feeding him properly?' cause all manner of doubts, worries, and guilt.

A child's appetite is generally a reflection of his rate of growth, and as growth varies greatly with the child's age, there are obviously considerable variations in appetite. Put very simply, growth is fastest at birth, remains very fast in the first two years, then becomes slow and steady from three to ten years, before the growth spurt of adolescence. Growth doesn't increase steadily with age, and neither does appetite. This may come as a surprise to you, but when you consider the variations in normal growth, it is really only to be expected.

Any consideration of growth must start at birth, and

birth weights are always of great interest. Cards that parents send out to announce a birth never mention length, or size of feet, but always have a space for the proud parents to enter their child's weight. The largest ever baby born alive, incidentally, weighed in at 20 lb 8 oz (9.299 kg) and measured 23 in (58 cm) in length.

A child's size at birth is affected by two main factors – his inheritance, and the environment in his mother's womb before birth. Tall parents tend to have larger babies, and racial factors have an influence too – although sometimes it is difficult to unravel how much the differences in size of children of different races is due to their genes or their environment. The regions boasting the largest average birth weights are Lapland (3.3 kg) and the Arctic (where Russian Eskimos have an average birth weight of 3.48 kg), presumably because of their cold climates.

In the United Kingdom and the USA the average birthweight for babies is just over 7 lb (or 3.2 kg). However in all discussions of weight it is absolutely essential to be wary of averages. All the average means is that half of all babies born will be 7 lb or less, and half will be 7 lb or more. A 6 lb baby is usually every bit as normal as a 7 lb one, and as I consider the whole question of normal growth, I will show you how to base your predictions of growth accurately on your own child – not on a mythical average.

On an international scale, malnutrition is one of the most important factors to affect birth weight. Women in underdeveloped countries with poor nutrition have smaller babies than women in countries with better nutrition. In addition there is a social class variation, with lower social class parents having lighter babies. There is a similar link with intelligence, and also with the mother's weight before the pregnancy. Large babies tend to be born to taller and heavier mothers, and older mothers. If a mother is diabetic, has diabetes in her family, or is going to become diabetic much later in her life, then she is likely to have a large baby. For some strange reason, babies born in March, April or May tend to be larger than average, while June, July, and August births are smaller.

There are several important reasons why babies are born smaller, and one – at least – is completely avoidable. Mothers who smoke during pregnancy have babies an average of 6 oz (170 g) lighter than non-smokers. Smoking causes the blood vessels in the placenta to contract and less blood reaches the baby. As a result their nutrition is not so good, and this particularly affects the brain. It has been conclusively shown that the children of smoking mothers are less intelligent than those of their non-smoking colleagues. Smoking before pregnancy has no effect on the baby. Even as late as school age it has been shown that children born to smokers are significantly smaller than those born to non-smokers.

Other maternal factors which lead to low birth weight babies are high blood pressure during pregnancy, chronic kidney disease, multiple pregnancy, certain infections, certain types of drug taking, and radiation. If the mother's diet is very poor this understandably leads to poor growth for the foetus as well.

In the first few days of life, most babies lose weight – usually around one ounce a day for the first five days. This weight is regained by day ten, and then the average baby gains about 6 to 7 oz (170–200 gm) each week until a 7 lb baby will have reached about 21 lb (9.5 kg) at one year of age.

You may well have heard such figures enshrined in the saying that 'an average baby doubles his birth weight by six months and trebles it in a year'. This sort of saying can cause all sorts of anxiety, unless you remember the dreaded word 'average'. For the typical 'average' 7 lb baby this saying is certainly tme, but it does not apply for smaller or larger babies. For instance a 6 lb baby will double its weight in three months and treble it in six months. You will see this clearly from the growth charts later in the chapter. Similarly an 8 lb baby who trebled his weight in a year would be dreadfully fat. Parents of either of these children would possibly get very worried if their child didn't seem to be following 'the rules'. Please remember the rules are only a very rough guideline for the parents of 'average' children.

Remembering this warning, it is fair to say that the average child will gain 7 lb (3.17kg) in his second year and 5 lb (2.27 kg) in the third. You can see immediately that growth has slowed right down from the initial growth spurt, and appetite will decrease to match this. The various ante-natal factors affecting growth are still having an important effect in the first couple of years, which makes it difficult to judge a child's final height until they are two to three years old. As a very rough guide it is possible to say that the height of the adult will be twice that of the child at two years, give or take 2 cm.

The slow rate of growth in the second year (only 1–2 oz, or 28–57 g per week) means that it is pointless weighing your child frequently during this stage. Few scales are accurate enough to measure such small changes, and three-monthly weighing and measuring is certainly adequate. For younger children the frequency with which you weigh your child is very much up to you. For most parents whose children seem happy and healthy very frequent weighing is hardly necessary. Health visitors or doctors should arrange regular checks to keep an eye on growth and development, but if you are particularly concerned, anxious or interested in your child's growth and want to weigh and measure him weekly then may I offer a word of warning. Children rarely grow in a steady way. Some weeks they gain a lot, and other weeks the weight gain stops. In other words, if you plotted weight on a graph it would go up in steps. Now, the more frequently you weigh your child the more chance there is that you will come across the 'no-gain' flat part of the step, and this may well worry you. The parent who weighs less often will only see the average gains, and not the irrelevant steps. I would certainly consider it well worthwhile to weigh and measure your child accurately every six months from birth to maturity and record it on a growth chart of the kind provided later in this chapter.

Weighing can be important, particularly if you are worried about your child for some other reason, but don't let it become an obsession. Continually weighing and comparing weights with other parents may even lead to an element of parental competition which can result in obese babies. If your child is healthy and developing well, don't get worried by what his weight does in any given week. Similarly if he has gained weight satisfactorily, but doesn't seem 'right' in some other way, then don't be falsely reassured. Get him checked over.

After the fairly slow growth rate of the second and third years, his weight will continue to increase comparatively slowly until he reaches adolescence. However, as well as this slow and steady growth, the child's proportions change fairly dramatically too. A newborn baby's head (and brain) is very large in proportion to the rest of the body. In the first year of life the head circumference enlarges from an average of 13 in (33 cm) to 18 in (45.7 cm). To see how the relative proportions of the body change compare this 5 in (12.7 cm) of growth with the total growth of 3 in (7.62 cm) over the next eleven years. While at birth the head is a quarter the size of the trunk, in the adult it is only one eighth of the size. In addition the size of the limbs in relation to the rest of the body changes very significantly.

These changing proportions affect how the child looks. A one-year-old who has just started walking may look a very odd creature with his large head, bow legs, and protuberant abdomen. He looks fine when crawling, but most out of proportion when standing. Similarly by the age of two or three he will have slimmed down and looks far more like a normal child. During this slimming-out phase, many parents get worried that their child is 'skinny' and decide he needs extra food. Don't fall into this trap. If you consult the growth charts you will see he almost certainly isn't too thin at all, but you may have got so used to your chubby-looking toddler that he looks far too slender when his proportions change.

The next major growth spurt arrives, of course, with adolescence. In general girls mature some two-and-a-half years earlier than boys, and have their spurt of growth much sooner. Nevertheless, they tend to end up an average of 6 in (15 cm) shorter than their brothers. The first sign of puberty in girls is usually development of the breasts. Don't worry if one side develops before the other. This is extremely common. The usual order of development is then pubic hair, underarm hair, development of the genitals, and finally menstruation. By the time menstruation occurs, the maximum growth rate has almost always passed. Quite frequently tall girls enter puberty early, and following an early spurt growth ceases. In fact they frequently end up shorter than their contemporaries.

The usual order of development for boys is the appearance of pubic hair, followed by enlargement of the genitals, the breaking of the voice, and then growth of the beard and underarm hair.

This consideration of the growth and development of an 'average' child has assumed that he had an adequate diet and favourable environment in which to grow. But both severe malnutrition and serious illness can hinder growth and the longer these go on the more severe the effect. However if normal growth is affected by illness, there is usually a catch-up phase when the child recovers. During this, growth accelerates rapidly, and then when the child is back on his original course it slows back down to normal. Obviously such a process cannot happen in the presence of significant malnutrition.

Other factors affect growth, some more easily explained than others. For instance, growth is faster in spring and slower in autumn, while weight gain is fastest in the winter – presumably a combination of the child eating more and doing less. I will consider other causes of poor weight gain and growth in Chapter 7.

Over recent years children have certainly been growing more. In Glasgow, for example, children are reaching a height 10 cm taller than they were some sixty years ago, presumably linked with improvements in nutrition over the years. Over the past thirty years, the average height of young people in China has increased at a rate of almost 1 inch every ten years. A 1979 survey of 20,000 students in sixteen provinces showed that the boys were 5.6 cm (2¼ in) taller than those in 1955, with a similar increase for girls. This improvement has been put down to the increased quantity of protein eaten by the average Chinese child.

If you do have a child who is considerably taller than average, then it is particularly important to bear in mind his actual age, rather than the age he looks. It is terribly easy, and very unfair, to treat a tall six-year-old as a nine-year-old and expect him to behave accordingly. If he doesn't, you will probably get cross and he will have every reason to suspect that you are being unreasonable. I have experience of this myself. My daughter has, for several years, been much taller than her school friends. One day, I well recall getting very irritated with her and told her 'be your age'. With more insight than she realized, she replied, 'But I am!' She was right. I was expecting standards of behaviour from her that I would never have demanded of a smaller child. The tall child can become very self-conscious at the best of times: it is vital that parents don't undermine what confidence the child has.

The majority of tall children have 'tallness' in the family. If the parents themselves aren't tall, it is likely that uncles, aunts, and grand-parents are. There are also a number of rare syndromes, such as gigantism, Marfan's syndrome, and Kleinefelter's syndrome, but with all these you should spot that growth is not as you would predict on the growth charts.

Growth charts are an absolutely essential tool in the assessment of growth, and are the only way of accurately judging how your child's height and weight relate to each other, and to expectations. The growth charts reproduced here were first developed by Professor Tanner and his colleagues at London's Institute of Child Health, and similar charts are used by doctors throughout the world.

The reason a chart is essential is quite simple. A single measurement of your child's weight and height is completely useless. Let us say, for example, that you measure your six-year-old and find that he is 110 cm tall. By itself, that information is meaningless. It cannot tell you whether his height is correct for his age and potential, or if he should be 120 cm and is failing to grow sufficiently, or even if he should be 100 cm and is very tall for his age.

What is required is a series of measurements taken at different ages. This will show how his growth is changing and will give some idea of whether he is still growing at the same speed as he has done in the past.

However, even this alone can be misleading. We have

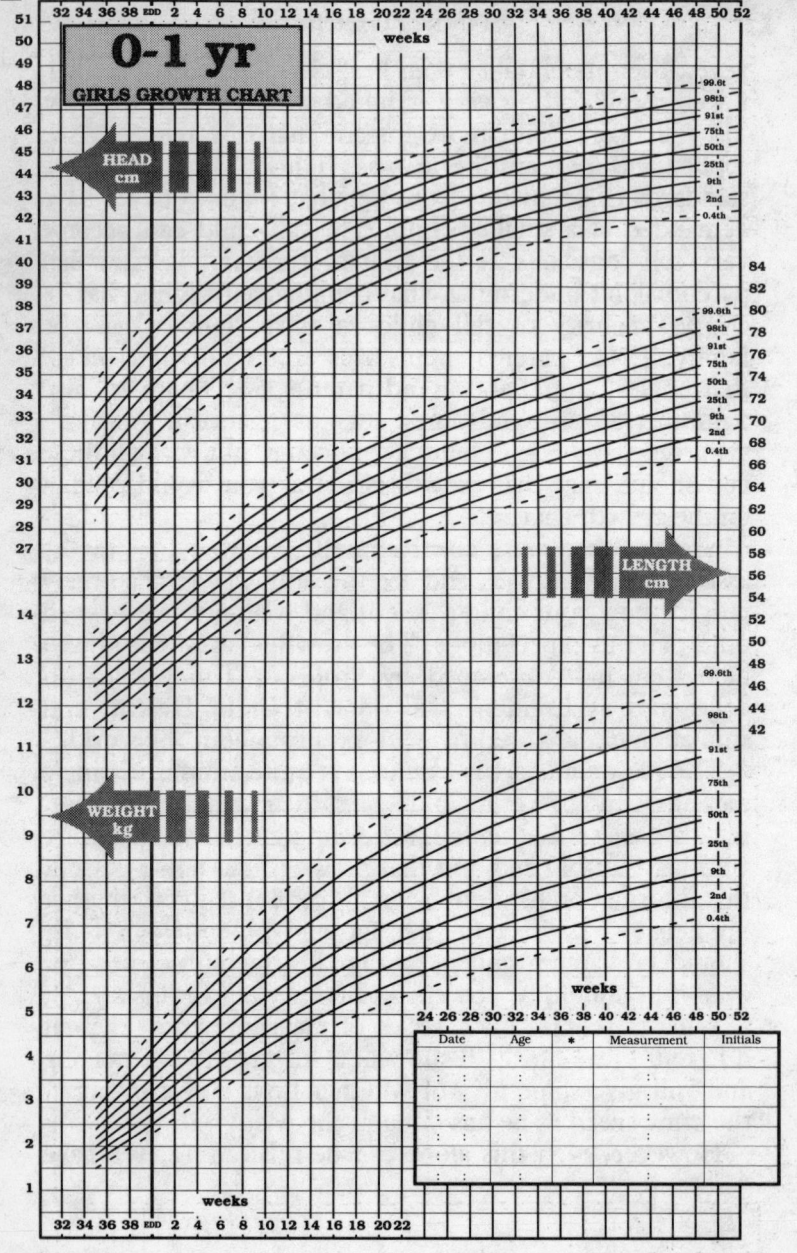

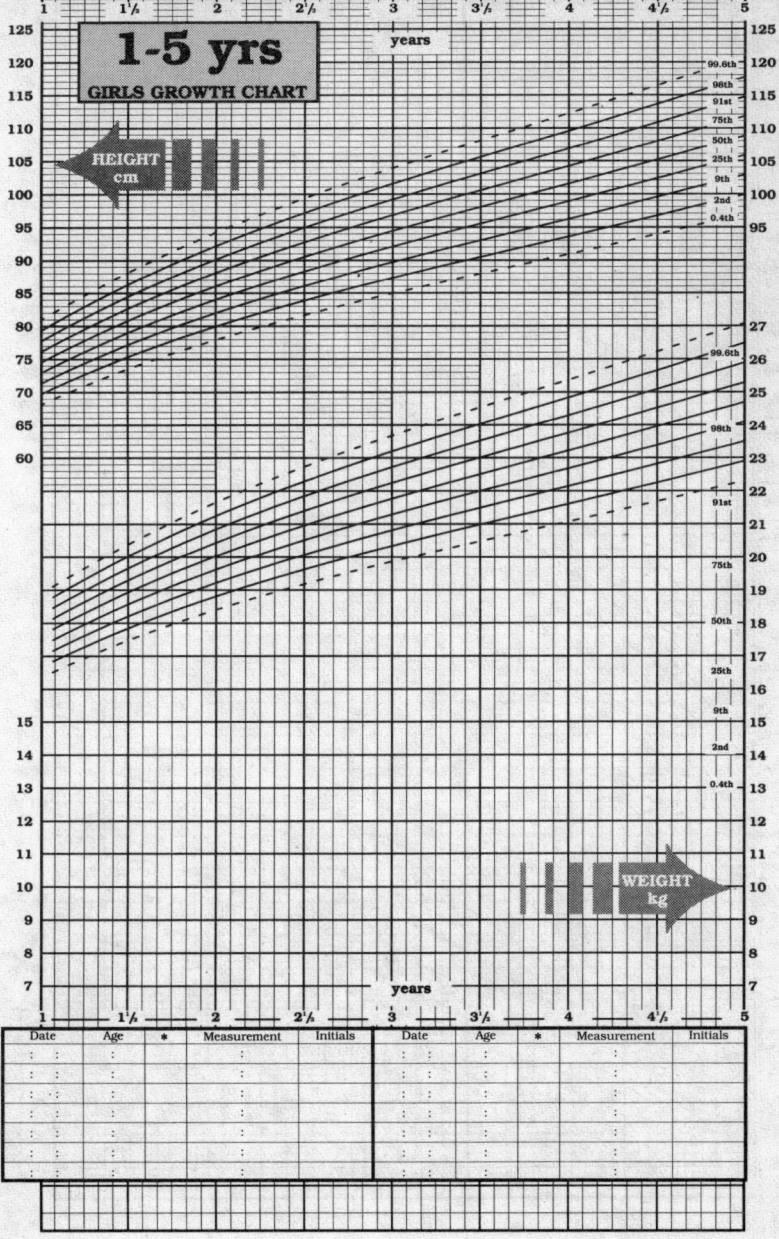

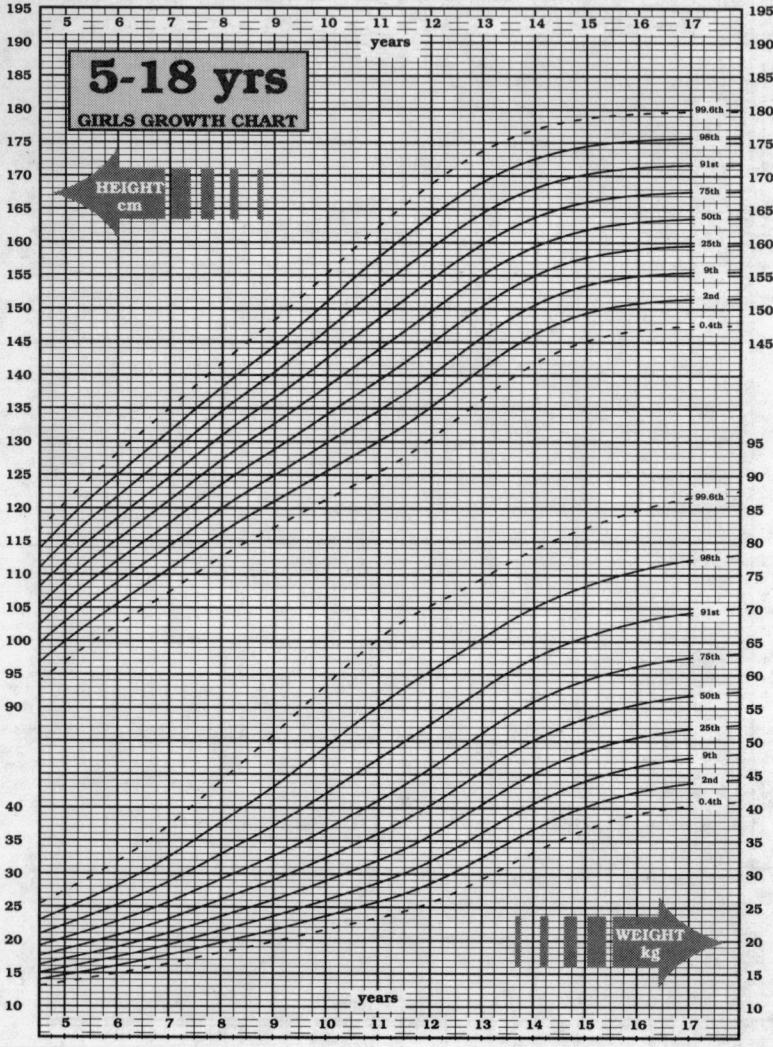

5-18 yrs

GIRLS GROWTH CHART

HEIGHT cm

WEIGHT kg

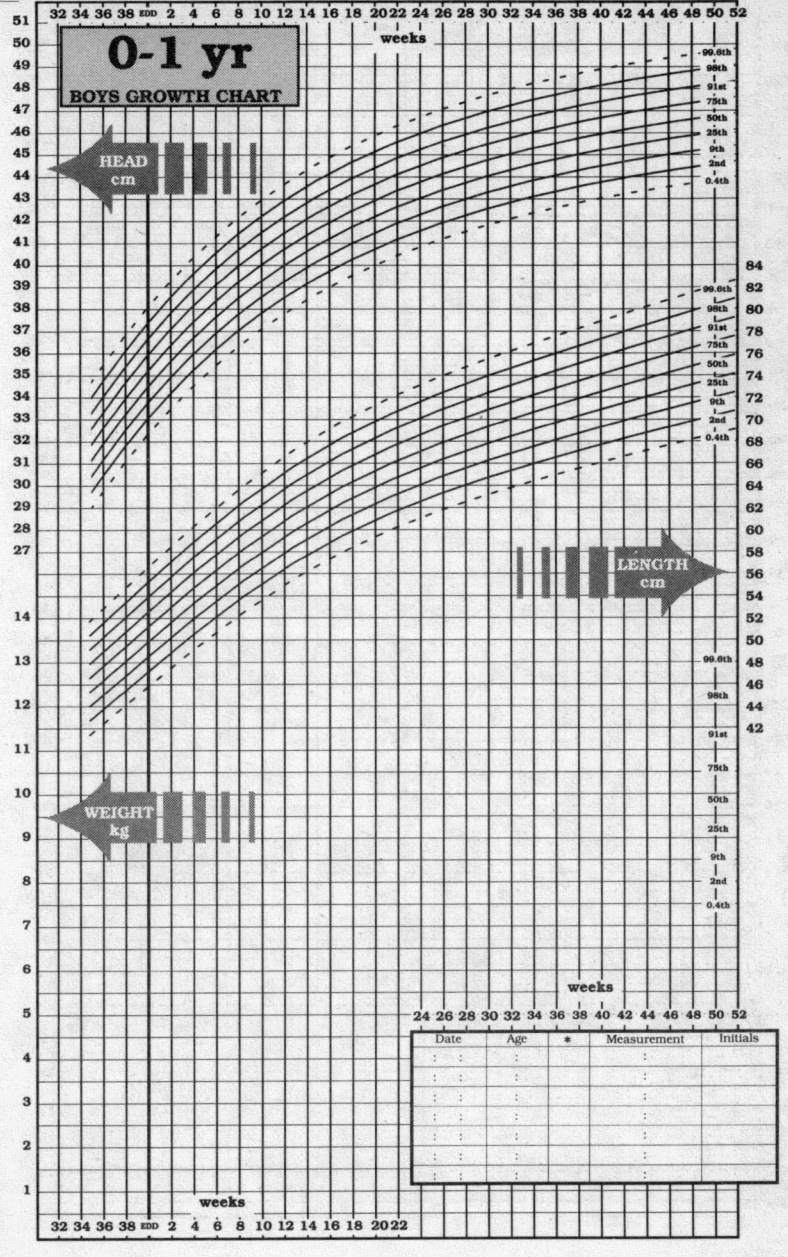

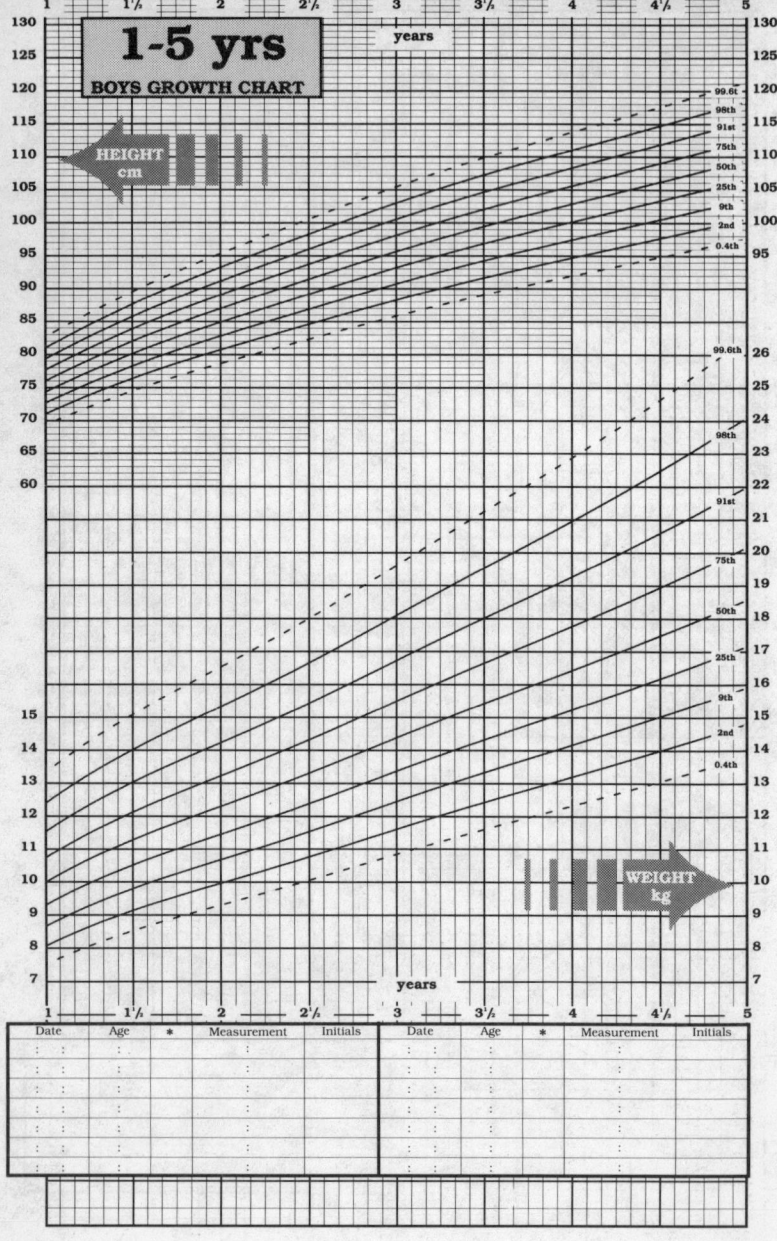

1-5 yrs
BOYS GROWTH CHART

years

HEIGHT cm

99.6th
98th
91st
75th
50th
25th
9th
2nd
0.4th

99.6th

98th

91st

75th

50th

25th

9th
2nd

0.4th

WEIGHT kg

years

Date	Age	*	Measurement	Initials	Date	Age	*	Measurement	Initials
: :	:		:		: :	:		:	
: :	:		:		: :	:		:	
: :	:		:		: :	:		:	
: :	:		:		: :	:		:	
: :	:		:		: :	:		:	

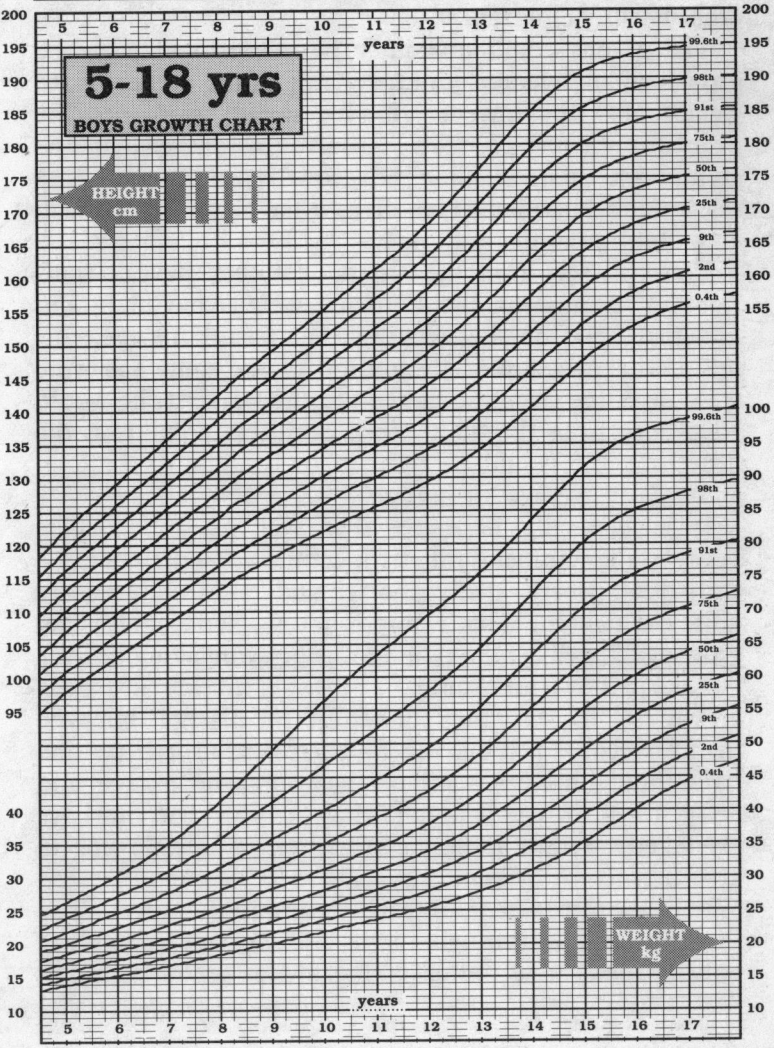

already seen how growth varies at different ages, being much faster in the first year, for example, than in the fourth year. To judge how a given child is growing, we therefore need to be able to compare him or her with other healthy children.

The graphs could obviously be overprinted with the growth of an 'average' child, starting at the average birth weight of 7 lb. However, I have already explained the problems of using averages. To solve this, rather than just giving one 'normal' line of growth on the graph, a selection is provided. This gives a far better comparison with children of the same age.

You will see from the charts that they have various 'centiles' printed on them. If you weigh your child and find that he is on the twentieth centile for his age, this means that if a hundred children of the same age were stood in a line from the lightest to the heaviest, he would be twenty from the 'light' end. Similarly a child on the fiftieth centile would be right in the middle of the line, and exactly average for his age.

It is generally accepted that weights and heights between the tenth and ninetieth centile are quite normal – and, don't worry, many shorter and taller children are quite normal too. What is important is when a child is not growing along a centile that he was growing along before.

Take a boy, for example, who all his life has been growing along the ninetieth centile for his age, but who then is recorded as having fallen to the fiftieth centile. Even though his size is still on the average for his age, and he is still growing, it is not what the charts would have predicted for him and an explanation of this slowing in growth must be looked for.

In other words, a child usually continues to grow along the same centile throughout his life, but the centile can only be determined after taking a number of measurements. However, there are a few exceptions. Many children have what is called delayed maturation – in other words they tend to grow along the tenth centile until late in adolescence when they suddenly shoot up and end up at a size far greater than one would have predicted from their earlier measurements. Children who do this usually have a parent or other close relative whose growth was delayed in a similar way. If this is the case then there is no cause for concern.

In Chapters 7 and 8 I will be considering abnormal growth in more detail, when considering the problems of the underweight and overweight child. I will also be giving more detailed calculations for working out your child's likely height as an adult.

Before leaving growth charts for the moment one final point needs making. Quite simply, when you weigh and measure your child, mind you do it accurately. If you use a cheap pair of bathroom scales, make sure they are zeroed before use, and preferably use the same scales for each weighing. When measuring height, do not try and do it directly with a tape measure. Instead stand your child against the wall, heels flat on the floor. Make sure he is looking straight ahead, then place a flat object such as a book on his head and mark on the wall at the level of the book. You can then measure from the floor to the mark. It is interesting (and fun) to leave the marks there as a permanent record of growth.

When you do plot growth on the charts you will need to compare weight and height. If he is gaining weight faster than height, then he is getting fat. If there is virtually no growth in height over a six-month period, re-measure after another couple of months. If there is still no growth take the charts and measurements to your doctor for his or her advice. Very occasionally treatment will be needed.

Finally, don't get too obsessed with all these measurements. It is most unlikely that there is anything seriously wrong with a happy, energetic child. You will almost certainly be able to sit back and watch such a child grow with pleasure and pride.

4

Mealtimes and Manners

'Mealtimes have become a dreadful strain. Every meal is more like a battle. I thought families were supposed to enjoy eating together. That will be the day!'

Mother of four-year-old girl

Good nutrition consists of far more than simply food in adequate quantities. Recently more and more evidence has shown that the frequency and timing of meals is just as important for long-term health. Very many adults go for long periods without anything other than a snack and then have a huge meal in the evening. This is far from ideal. The more that your intake of food is spread through the day, the better – and this applies even more to your children.

However, the actual timing of meals is far more a matter of habit than of any biological law. There are variations from society to society, with different cultures having quite different expectations as to what and when a meal should be. Take the example of the tea-break. In any office, shop, or other work place the timing of the tea-break follows a set routine. If, for example, everyone is used to having a cup of tea at four, and one day it is delayed to half past four, there will inevitably be numerous comments like 'I'm dying for a cup of tea. How much longer must we wait?' Obviously no one is really going to suffer from the wait, and yet the habit can be so ingrained that the delay makes people feel they are genuinely suffering.

As far as your children are concerned two main rules are worth bearing in mind. Try to develop a regular mealtime routine, having meals at approximately the same time each day whenever possible. However, remember that many children – particularly toddlers – simply cannot digest a large meal at one sitting. As we will see in the next chapter, this is often a cause of apparent food refusal. A child who is offered too much food at once is quite right to refuse to eat some of it – whatever its parents might think!

Toddlers, as I said, are far better having small meals with snacks in between – particularly if the snack is reasonably nutritious. Problems arise if the snack is filling, but not nutritious, as the next meal will be refused as the child feels full. Inevitably a vicious circle will soon start up and worsen your problems. Because your child is full he doesn't want his next meal, and because he doesn't eat the meal he needs another snack shortly afterwards. I will consider snacks and 'between-meal-eating' again in Chapter 6.

The traditional pattern of meals in most Western cultures is still 'three square meals' a day. Of these, most parents see the midday and evening meal as the most important. Generally far less concern is shown if breakfast is missed than if one of the later meals is refused. Interestingly there is wide variation in what different meals are called, even within a relatively small area. To some people 'dinner' is the midday meal. To others it is the evening meal. For some, 'supper' is a light snack at bedtime, whilst others see 'supper' as the main evening meal. There are also locally specific variations. In parts of Eastern England, farm workers have a main meal at around 11 o'clock in the morning which is known as 'dockie'.

Such variations in eating habits are fascinating, and – if nothing else – go to show that mealtimes are far from being biological laws. Mealtimes are largely matters of cultural habit, and while children eventually have to learn to adapt to the society they live in, it may be reassuring to know that their reluctance to eat at certain times may simply be because they haven't yet learnt that this is how your family does things.

Incidentally, the varying names and times of meals do prompt one important caveat. If a doctor tells you to give your child a medicine before meals, or before supper, then check exactly what he means. His definition of 'supper' may be different from yours, and his 'before meals' may mean four times a day – before breakfast, lunch, afternoon tea and the evening meal. It is vital that doctors and parents make sure they are speaking the same language.

The meal that is usually given the least consideration, and yet which matters a very great deal, is breakfast. In America it has been estimated that three-quarters of families do not eat breakfast together, and in up to half of all families, one or more people regularly miss breakfast. In about four families out of ten, the parents have nothing to do with the child's breakfast.

Of course, the trouble with breakfast is when it happens. Few people feel at their best in the morning. Adults may have to go out to work. Children have to go to school. Hair needs combing. Teeth need brushing. School books get lost. Tempers get frayed. No wonder a calm, relaxed, enjoyable breakfast together is something of a rarity, and the instant breakfast so popular. A bowl of cereal can be prepared and eaten almost without the eater needing to wake up.

Much abuse is thrown at the breakfast food manufacturers by some of the 'health food' fanatics. Certainly some cereals do contain too much sugar, and some are nutritionally far from ideal, but they are all far, far better than nothing. For many families, the choice at breakfast is a bowl of cereal or nothing at all, and the cereal wins every time.

Of course, if you can find the time now and again to prepare your family a really delicious hot breakfast, or other foods such as home-baked bread or rolls, then that is ideal. Indeed, I would encourage you to do so as often as possible. Children take many of their attitudes to meals from their parents, and if your attitude is that breakfast is a nuisance that needs to be got over as quickly as possible, then don't be surprised if your children feel the same. However if you eat a decent breakfast yourself, your children will learn from your example.

Few meals seem to have such a limited repertoire of foods, and yet there is absolutely no reason for this. Most people find it hard to think beyond cereal, toast, bacon, and eggs, but this is only habit. When he was six, my son was going through a phase of refusing everything we offered at breakfast. Eventually we asked him what he did want. Without hesitation he said, 'Chicken soup and pork pie.' It sounded revolting, and our initial reaction was to tell him not to be so silly. But why? Only convention dictates that chicken soup is not acceptable at breakfast and is acceptable four hours later at lunch. For a week he had soup every day, then tired of it, and changed to something else. A battle was saved, he had a thoroughly nutritious breakfast, and we were taught a valuable lesson. Use your imagination when it comes to breakfast time, and have a look at any cook books that offer unusual and different breakfast suggestions.

When it comes to cereals, do try and avoid the presweetened ones if you can. Many of the sugar-coated cereals contain a tablespoon of sugar or more in a 1 oz serving. Try hiding the sugar bowl too. Sugar is a habit that is easy to acquire, and much harder to break. Avoid the very high fibre breakfasts, such as All-Bran, for the very young as they are too filling for them. Finally, if you really find thinking about breakfast too much for you to cope with first thing in the morning – then think about it the night before.

Why this accent on breakfast time? You may feel that as the other main meals are generally much bigger, they are far more important. However, breakfast *is* a child's most important meal. To play, or to learn, effectively, they need to have eaten something in the morning. A study in America over a ten-year period showed that schoolchildren who skipped breakfast became careless and inattentive in the late morning, but their work improved dramatically if breakfast was eaten. In the UK school timetables for those up to the age of eleven are planned on the assumption that children are at their most attentive in the morning, and the more important subjects tend to be concentrated then.

Many teachers have told me that they notice some children's work improves after the mid-morning 'break' when a snack is eaten. This is usually the first food these children have eaten that day. If how your child does at play, play-school, or school, concerns you – then please make sure he gets his breakfast.

What of the other meals? In Chapter 1 I discussed the general nutritional guidelines that are recommended today, and in the next chapter I will be offering suggestions on what to do if your child simply doesn't want to know! However, don't forget that there is more to mealtimes than simply providing food. Mealtimes are a social occasion too. They are often the only time that a family all sits down together and the importance of this must never be underestimated.

For many families, the only possible meal when everyone can regularly eat together is the evening meal. If there are very young children, they may need feeding earlier – before the breadwinner arrives home – but everyone else can enjoy their food together. Unfortunately the evening is probably the worst time to have one's main meal, but in the United Kingdom and America, work and school practices frequently don't allow families to get together at midday. The French have, for generations, believed in family meals at midday – and as a result the whole nation seems to shut down for a couple of hours at lunchtime. Their priorities are different; impractical for many people, but they have much to commend them.

The extent to which mealtimes are social occasions varies quite remarkably by social class. John and Elizabeth Newson in their splendid study of four-year-olds and their families in Nottingham showed this very clearly. In this survey, the parents of four-year-olds were asked a large number of questions about their attitudes to child-rearing, and problems that they faced. In one of those questions parents were asked if they minded in what order children ate their foods. If you think about it, there can be no nutritional reason why such an order is important. However, 81 per cent of the professional-class parents did mind if food was eaten in 'the wrong order'. Of working-class parents, however, a majority (58 per cent) did not mind at all.

The Newsons attributed this to the greater formality of mealtimes as one ascends the class scale. If a meal is a family gathering when everyone sits down together to exchange their news, then a set pattern of eating is expected to be followed. For many working-class families, each person sits down as they arrive in from work. There is no pattern to be disrupted, and the purpose of the meal is seen quite differently.

The whole question of table manners needs considering in the same light. There are no rights and wrongs – just differences. Children should learn what is expected of them in their family situation.

Take the intriguing question of talking at mealtimes. The Newsons, when they looked at the replies to their questions about talking at table, concluded that for most working-class families eating is a serious business and 'there's plenty of time to talk afterwards'. The middle classes, however, see meals as social occasions when news and views should be exchanged. The child who doesn't talk in such a family might be considered surly and rude, and yet born into a different family such behaviour might be considered ideal.

Table manners concern all parents, though the Newsons found middle-class mothers particularly concerned. This is understandable if meals are seen as social occasions. In addition, middle-class families tend to entertain more frequently at mealtimes and there is consequently more concern about being 'shown up' by children with poor table manners.

One mother wrote to me, 'I really don't know what to do with Joanne. She can eat beautifully – if I nag her about it. If I don't, she messes with her food, sits slumped with her elbow on the table, and looks a real mess. I don't want to nag her as it casts a cloud over the whole meal, but I hate to think what other people must think of her when she eats at their houses.'

Children, of course, are remarkably devious creatures. The child who never behaves in his own house will frequently be a little angel when visiting friends or relatives. 'Please' and 'Thank you' and 'May I get down' get said without any prompting. Many are the parents who look disbelieving when told how well their child behaves at table, when the same child behaves like an untrained chimpanzee in his own home.

Perhaps the only important rule is for parents to behave at table as they would wish their child to behave. Example often has far more effect than nagging. Families who don't believe in reading at the table should ban father from reading the newspaper as well as children from reading comics. It is illogical to allow one and not the other. Similarly, if you don't want your child to have his elbows on the table, then check where yours are first. It can be embarrassing.

Pre-school children tend to be somewhat erratic and messy in their eating, and too many battles over table manners will make mealtimes even less enjoyable. However by school age your child should be able to be more sociable in his eating. Try not to rush things, however. To allow him to finger-feed one day, and to ban it the next, is asking for trouble. Slow gentle encouragement, coupled with good examples from his elders, will pay far more dividends. Try making at least one meal a week really special. The weekend is an ideal time for this welcome change for everyone from the hurriedly served and snatched meal in the kitchen. Lay the table 'formally', possibly asking your child to make some special decoration for the table centre. There are all sorts of little tricks that will make the meal special – whether it is paper napkins, a special drink with or before the meal, or whatever. Your child will feel a sense of privilege and excitement to be allowed to join in such a meal, and will almost certainly behave appropriately. As well as being enjoyable, he will learn how to behave on a special occasion, and will be far less likely to 'let you down' if he eats out.

In addition, the child who occasionally eats out with his

parents from an early age will not be overwhelmed by the experience. Unfortunately, until relatively recently in Britain, it has been quite disgraceful how little encouragement has been given to children to eat out with their parents, certainly compared to family restaurants in the USA and continental Europe.

However, improvements do seem to be filtering in. I have been privileged to be one of the judges of the 'Parent Friendly Campaign' since it first started. This campaign aims at encouraging businesses, such as shops, airports, and restaurants, to be more positive in their attitude towards parents and children. In our first year we were inundated with stories of dreadful service and indifferent attitudes. Typical were the pubs that advertise themselves with the words 'children welcome' and then force families to sit at rickety formica-topped tables in a cold and draughty outhouse.

At last things really do seem to be gradually improving, though. There are more genuinely family-orientated restaurants (often based on the excellent American restaurant chains), and families with young children aren't always treated nowadays as though they all had contagious diseases. For instance, one chain, Millers Kitchen, has been introducing family entertainment in the form of 'Jungle Bungles', purpose built indoor play barns specially designed for young children, and including giant slides and bouncy inflatables. Such a development would have been unheard of only a few years ago.

However, there are still problems. For instance, little imagination seems to be shown in the choice of food on offer. The typical 'Under Twelves Menu' usually has an exciting name ('Young Pirates Menu' or 'Spacefleet Canteen') and then offers a choice of burgers, sausages, fish fingers, baked beans, and chips. Perhaps it is now time for more enterprising ideas in the selection of children's menus. Perhaps marketing managers simply offer what they know has sold in the past, but they will never know what else children might choose if they never offer them the alternatives.

Many parents do worry a great deal over fast food. The damning label of 'junk food' has been applied to meals such as burgers and beans. However, such dishes are probably more nourishing than you think. The lack of fresh fruit in fast food restaurants is a sad omission, and the excess of fatty fried foods is to be regretted; however many nutritional specialists who have analysed 'junk foods' usually conclude that as long as they are not taken for every meal every day they could certainly be a lot worse.

One big fast food chain, McDonald's, has obviously become so concerned about their image with parents that they have produced a series of advertisements which list the nutritional composition in their milk shakes, french fries, and so on. Indeed, they also produce detailed leaflets and booklets which are available on request and compare the content of their foods with advised nutritional guidelines. The increasing interest in the quality and nutritional value of food has affected the manufacturers, and in the long run that has to be a good thing. Some hamburger chains, notably Wendy's, now offer a salad bar, and others are offering excellent pre-packaged salads, so there is clearly a change occurring. Foods such as salads do at least provide some of the variety that fast food outlets currently lack.

If your storecupboards at home are packed with fresh fruits, yogurts, wholemeal bread, fresh vegetables and so on, and you do not constantly rely on convenience foods and fried foods, then your child or adolescent will come to no harm choosing fast foods when he goes out. Fast foods are a relatively expensive way of eating, but as the occasional 'treat' you really need not worry too much. Whether it is pizza, burgers, fish and chips, or whatever does not really matter. Remember the guidelines I mentioned in Chapter 1 for your everyday eating, and bow to the fact that youngsters do love fast food and there's no escaping it occasionally. If you make your own copies of favourite fast food meals at home, then you can easily reduce the fat, shake a little less salt, and put the burger in a wholemeal bun. Oven-ready chips are certainly an improvement on ordinary deep frying, as the frying makes them almost twice as fatty. It also helps to make your chips as thick as possible. If a potato is cut up into lots of thin, stringy chips, its surface area is far greater than if it had been cut into thick chips. The greater the surface area, the greater the amount of fat in the final serving. 'Crinkle-cutting' also increases the fat content.

The one other significant advantage in making your own copies of fast foods is that you can add more variety. Offering a side salad, or giving fresh fruit as a dessert, will result in a much better all-round meal.

For many children, however, the one place where they do regularly eat away from their parents is at school. Until recently, school dinners provided the main cooked meal of the day for up to half of all school-age children. However regulations and benefits have changed.

Today, education authorities must make provision for meals 'as appears to be requisite' in the middle of the day, but they do not have any responsibility to provide a suitable main meal of the day. When it comes to charges, all pupils must be charged the same price for meals or other refreshments, unless they are entitled to free meals, and the only children who are now entitled to free school meals are those who are members of a family of a person receiving income support.

In the past there used to be fairly rigid guidelines as to

what nutrients should be provided by school meals. For example, it was recommended that one-third of daily energy needs, and half the daily protein requirement, should be provided by a school dinner. Such recommendations were fine on paper, and doubtless the required nutrients were put on the plate. In my school days, at least, many of them stayed there! They made their way straight to the waste bin, not making children grow at all.

In 1980 the Education Act in Britain allowed local authorities to charge what they wanted for school meals, and also abandoned any nutritional criteria. Now the schools have no obligation to provide food of any particular standard. Market forces rule.

This change has had many effects – not all of them entirely beneficial. There can be little doubt that reasonably nutritious food that children will eat and enjoy is preferable to extremely nutritious food that they leave on their plate. However, the whole question of payment for meals, however excellent their value, does pose problems. The very poor families will get free meals. The affluent families, who will probably eat well at home anyway, will pay for them willingly. There is however a group of children who would probably benefit from such meals whose parents earn just too much for them to get free meals, and who are reluctant to pay the price of the meal. There are many reasons for this reluctance, and not all of them are entirely logical. One parent told me that she couldn't afford to find the cash every day, particularly when she had food in the cupboard that she could send as a packed lunch 'and which doesn't cost me anything'. In other words she saw food that she had already paid for as being free. When we looked at what she had sent with her child to school, it had actually cost more than the school meal would have done. This problem of the organization of domestic budgeting is, I suspect, fairly common.

A survey of school children's eating habits published in the *British Medical Journal* found that children who relied on packed lunches or food they bought out of school got significantly lower nutritional value than they would have had from a school lunch. The most common food bought outside schools is, if course, chips. A bag of chips and a Coke cannot, by any possible definition, constitute an acceptable lunch for a school child day in day out.

As school meals increase in price more parents will inevitably turn to packed lunches for their children. If you do so please try and give a reasonable mixture of foods. Biscuits and crisps are not enough. Cheese, bread, fruit, meat or fish (as in sandwiches), are much better. Offer variety too. Would you want to eat a cheese sandwich *every* day? You can plan ahead too. Sandwiches can be frozen, depending on their contents – hard boiled eggs go very rubbery – and many mothers prepare a week's sandwiches at a time, freezing them, and then allowing the next day's supply to defrost overnight. It is possible to produce a packed lunch that is every bit as enjoyable and nutritious as a cooked meal, but it does take thought. There are plenty of cook books with good suggestions.

To encourage children to have school meals, many schools now provide a cafeteria-style service. Most secondary schools offer a choice of foods, though this is unusual in primary schools. A number of people responsible for the service throughout the country have told me that it would cease tomorrow if they no longer had a legal obligation to provide the free meals for the poorest children. The kitchens have to be there, and so the free meals protect the service for the others.

School meals services face tremendous problems when deciding what to offer in the way of foods. One organizer told me, 'If we provide chips every day, the parents complain. If we don't provide chips, the children go down to the nearest chip shop and buy chips there. We try and compromise by using polyunsaturated cooking oils, which at least means that our chips are probably better than the chip shop ones, but parents still complain.'

Another said, 'We keep being asked by parents to provide old-fashioned school meals. Meat and two vegetables with gravy. That sort of thing. If we do, the children either won't eat or won't buy it, or leave it on their plates. Surely it is better for us to provide fish fingers that they will eat, than liver which they won't?' I couldn't agree more.

Having said that, it cannot be denied that most school meals are ten years behind the times. They contain too little fibre, too much sugar, and too much fat. A survey carried out for the Inner London Education Authority confirmed that this was the case, but yet again they found that the school meals were still nutritionally more valuable than the usual alternatives.

Other absurd pressures on the school meals service act against healthy eating. Within the European Community there is an excess of dairy products – the so-called 'butter mountain'. As a result, one school meal organizer told me that whilst she was aware that she should offer less dairy fat in the meals, she received a greater subsidy for using full fat milk than skimmed milk in an attempt to reduce the dairy product surplus. The government really needs to decide if its responsibilities lie more with the nation's finances or its health.

I can only hope that the school meal service does continue for many years, as the prospect of children facing their morning lessons with no breakfast inside them, and their afternoon lessons with only a bag of chips to keep them going, doesn't fill me with delight. However, as costs rise, the number of children taking meals falls, and as the numbers fall, the costs rise. It's another vicious circle in which our children are the losers.

And what is actually happening to our children? In 1994, a fascinating study was published which looked in remarkable detail at the nutrition of a group of school-children aged 12 to 13 in Hackney, a socially deprived area in east London. Of the 149 pupils in the second year, 65 agreed to take part. The children were provided with scales to weigh their food, and they also kept a food diary for seven days – though it won't surprise any parent to hear that one third of the food diaries were incomplete! The children also agreed to provide blood samples, look-ing at both the level of iron and the level of cholesterol in their blood.

Many of the findings were fascinating. A third of the children ate nothing before starting school in the morning, only 20 per cent ate breakfast cereals regularly, and 74 per cent did not meet the recommended intake of fibre.

Lots of chips, sweets, and fizzy drinks were consumed, with the average number of portions of chips eaten being three per week for boys, and 3.6 for girls. Girls also ate more crisps – 5.8 bags per week, compared to 2.6 per week for boys.

When it came to fruit, over one in three had no fresh fruit during the week, and only a fifth had vegetables (other than potatoes) on a daily basis. The blood tests revealed a significantly low level of ferritin – which is linked with iron deficiency and anaemia – but – despite many of the horrors of the diet (85 per cent of the children were eating far too much fat), levels of cholesterol in the blood were generally low. More research is needed to look at the longer term effects on cholesterol levels.

Despite the fact that a significant number of the chil-dren were at risk of anaemia, I would certainly not recommend that all children should be given iron supplements 'just in case'. Another 1994 study, admittedly of much younger children than the Hackney school children, has shown that giving iron supplements to children who were not short of iron in their diet actually retarded their growth, and had no beneficial effects whatsoever.

One other particular occasion that causes parents great concern is the holiday abroad. It is not uncommon to see family cars waiting to board a ferry loaded high with every imaginable foodstuff. Evidently parents become very worried about the quality of food in foreign countries and feel safer taking their own.

Such an attitude would be more understandable if the family were off on a jaunt through Afghanistan or the Far East. It is less easy to grasp why food in France or Germany should pose such problems! If children do not get any taste of the country they are visiting they miss out on a lot. In fact, the provision for children in general is very much better in most other countries in Western Europe and in North America than it is in Great Britain. Excellent changing facilities for babies, well-designed play equipment at roadside picnic sites, and so forth, all indicate a far better acceptance of children than is often the case in the UK. Children are actually welcomed into many restaurants – an experience that may enormously surprise many British parents. In addition, many of the regulations with regard to food additives and colourings seem much stricter in countries such as France.

Of course, all the *usual* problems of food refusal can occur. The child who is reluctant to try new foods at home is equally likely to turn his nose up at them when abroad. However the basic childhood favourite foods – hamburgers, cheese, or eggs are good examples – are available almost everywhere and there is no need to fear your child will starve if you don't take enough food with you. Don't try and push new foods down your child. If he sees you enjoying them, more than likely he will eventually ask to try some. With our family, after a fortnight of refusing some local dish, the children would usually try it on the last day, declare it to be delicious, and be annoyed they had not sampled it before. After a few holidays abroad they learnt the lesson, and slowly became more adventurous.

There are a few simple rules of hygiene that I would strongly recommend when you are abroad. Wash or peel fruit before you eat it, particularly if you purchased it in a market where lots of people may have handled it. With young children, try and buy pre-wrapped ice-creams, rather than those that are doled out with an unhygienic and rarely washed scoop – a warning that applies equally in the U K. If you are in an area where the tap water is not drinkable, don't add ice to your otherwise safe drinks. Ice is rarely made from treated water in such areas. Finally, if you are flying take some sweets for the children to suck. Swallowing and sucking can prevent the misery of earache, and even the most 'anti-sweet' parent would be wise to relax the ban on such an occasion.

5

Food Refusal

*'I just don't know what to do next. Mealtime in our
house is one constant battle. I thought having children
was supposed to be a marvellously rewarding experience. When I look at my two turning up their noses at
yet another meal, then I go right off the whole idea of
being a parent. It's too late now, though.'*

Concern about children who are either faddy or eat very
little is tremendously common. In a study in America,
around one in five of three-year-olds was described as
having a very poor appetite, and more than one in ten had
very finicky tastes and ate an extremely limited diet. In
England, John and Elizabeth Newson found that 42 per
cent of the parents of four-year-olds in Nottingham were
concerned about their child's eating. For one-year-olds
the figure was only 10 per cent; clearly this worry increases
as children become toddlers and then preschoolers. There
are very good reasons for this, as we will see. Indeed faddy
eating can occasionally be a problem right up to school-
leaving age.

I have in front of me on my desk a thick file of letters
that I have received from parents. Over and over again
the same worries are repeated, and show the sheer frustration, concern, and even anger that this problem causes.
It is well worth quoting from a few of these.

The mother of one three-year-old wrote: 'For the past two years Laura has lived on cups of tea, biscuits and chocolate. Very occasionally she will eat scrambled egg or peanut butter sandwiches. But the mere mention of a meal and she either goes missing, bursts into tears, or has an urgent need for the toilet. When we do manage to sit her at the table she looks miserably at the meal and takes one mouthful, which she chews for ages then eventually spits it back on the plate.' (Incidentally, I certainly do not recommend that you offer children of this age tea or coffee as a drink, except for an occasional sip as a treat. Both are fairly strong stimulants, and can upset both behaviour and sleep patterns.)

Another mother wrote, with considerable feeling: 'I have a son aged nine and a half. As soon as he started mixed feeding he was fussy and would only eat two of the baby food dinners. By around eighteen months he suddenly started refusing food he would have eaten the day before. If we told him he must eat it, he said he felt sick. When we eventually said, "You won't be sick – eat it" – he was promptly sick. I was always asking doctors and health visitors how to get him to eat and they just said, "He's healthy – he'll come to it one day." I didn't believe a word of it.'

One of the most interesting letters came from a thirty-one-year-old lady who could look back at the problem from the child's point of view. She wrote: 'I have always hated potatoes. My mother used to try and disguise them by mashing them up with tomato ketchup, etc. I used to heave when forced to eat mash. My schooldays were made an absolute misery. Many an afternoon was spent in the Head's office with cold potatoes and pudding in front of me. To this day I will not eat potatoes.

'Very understandably,' she concluded, 'I feel very strongly indeed about the problem of forcing children to eat something they really hate.' It's easy to see why.

So – faddy eaters and food refusers are a common, important, and worrying problem. Why is this, and who has the problem, the parent or the child?

Faddy eating is a problem that is virtually unknown in very poor societies or families. If a child literally has no choice but 'eat it up, or starve' then he will eat. However, in the majority of Western families there is massive choice of which children are acutely aware. If television advertisements have taught him there are delicious and exciting convenience foods on the market, then his parents cannot really pretend otherwise. Breakfast cereals are a classic example. My children always seem to want any cereal other than the one they are offered.

Food refusal only very rarely goes so far as to cause severe malnourishment. Anorexia nervosa, a relatively rare problem in itself, is usually more often a problem of adolescents than young children and is dealt with later in the book. However the average faddy eater just will not eat what the parents want him to eat when the parents choose. Food refusal does not go so far as to endanger life. After all, children are born with an appetite that makes sure they don't starve. Unfortunately they are also born with an instinct to rebel if forced to something they don't want to do.

If faddy eaters don't actually come to any major harm, why do parents get so worried about the problem? I suspect that there are at least two main reasons, and numerous minor ones. There is genuine worry that a child's diet will be deficient in some way, and the child will not grow up as 'big and strong' as he should. There is also a worry about discipline. A child's refusal to eat is often seen as something which parents should be firm about.

After all, mothers often spend a very great deal of time preparing food. To have one's work rejected is always hurtful and upsetting and it is very hard to let it pass. Food also costs money, and for a child to leave a meal untouched is understandably seen as wasteful.

As often happens with such worries the issue may become complicated by other people. Granny may come to stay and make comments about how little her grand-child eats. Questions like 'Are you sure he's all right? He looks dreadfully thin,' and 'Look at how all his ribs are showing. Have you taken him to the doctor?' often make the parent feel worried, imcompetent, guilty, and angry.

Of course, the child cannot lose throughout all this. While granny stays he will either eat – in which case she will be able to say, 'See – he eats for me. You ought to be firmer' – or he doesn't, which goes to make granny even more concerned.

Other friends and parents may aggravate the situation too, with their comments on how little trouble their own children are. If this happens to you, remind yourself that over four out of ten parents share your worries, so you are in good company.

To consider these various worries, let us take them one at a time. It is quite easy to forget why you are worried and cross if your child will not eat. Next time you find you are having an argument because he won't eat up his carrots, for example, ask yourself precisely why you are so keen that he should. Is it because you think carrots are essential to his diet? They are not. As we saw in Chapter 1, very few foods are absolutely essential. If your child doesn't like certain foods it really is comparatively easy to give the nutrients in another way. I will return to this topic again shortly.

Perhaps you feel he should eat up his carrots purely as a matter of discipline. In other words, he should eat them because you have said so. Think about it. Is it really worth having a battle over such a trivial matter? It could be said of older children that if they like the foods their parents like then they are fine, but if they don't they are faddy. Is this what you are saying? Is it fair?

You may feel that his not eating carrots could be a sign of some illness or other. Finally, you may be concerned at the whole problem of waste. How many parents have told their children – 'Eat it up. Half the world is starving, and they would give anything for your meal.' It may be true, but it can hardly make sense to the child, and in practical terms it is nonsense too.

When you have decided just what it is about your child's eating habits that worries you, you can look in more depth at how justified those worries are.

Will he come to harm?

In Chapter 1, I spent a great deal of time explaining how remarkably – and surprisingly – unusual it is for a child to go short of essential nutrients. It is, however, important that children do at least have the chance of eating reasonably nutritious food.

Back in the 1930s, the paediatrician Clara Davis conducted a number of fascinating studies into children's diets. Quite simply, she allowed young children on a paediatric ward to select their own diet for several months. These children were allowed to feed themselves with whatever they wanted out of a wide range of wholesome foods, such as milk, fruit, eggs, vegetables, and so on. The food was put within reach, and they helped themselves with their fingers. No one tried to persuade them to eat one food or another, and if supplies of one food were finished, a fresh portion was put out.

Her findings showed two things quite clearly. Firstly,

and in the absence of adult attempts to control the infants' food intake, they grew well and were fit and healthy. Indeed, no stomach upsets at all happened during the time of the study, and when the 36,000 meals had all been analysed it was found that each child had balanced their diet perfectly. Davis went so far as to suggest 'the existence of some innate, automatic mechanism for its accomplishment.'

As well as this natural balancing, she also found that the children's diets varied quite remarkably. 'Tastes changed unpredictably.' 'Meals were a dietician's nightmare.' For instance, one child ate five eggs at one sitting, and others would occasionally go overboard for one food for a while, and then not touch it for days. Doesn't this sound just like the experience of most parents?

But this was the 1930s. Would the same thing happen in the 1990s, with all the changes in diet, discipline, advertising, junk food, and so on? A further study, published in 1991, was very reassuring. The researchers measured in detail the energy intake of fifteen young children, from 2 to 5 years of age, on six days. For each of the six days of the study, they calculated the energy intake of the various meals and snacks, and the total daily energy intake.

As in the earlier study, the children's intake at individual meals was highly variable, but the mean total daily energy intake stayed relatively constant. The researchers concluded that 'although children's food consumption is highly variable from meal to meal, daily energy intake is relatively constant, because children adjust their energy intake at successive meals.' Indeed, in most cases, high energy intake at one meal was followed by low energy intake at the next, and vice versa.

Not only is this sort of research enormously reassuring for parents, but these results have very real practical implications. Because many parents assume that their child cannot adequately regulate their food intake, watching with disbelief the differences from meal to meal, they often try to coerce their child to finish food that he or she doesn't want. This can be with bribes, or threats, or whatever. Such persuasion is more than likely going to be counterproductive. Indeed, attempts by parents to control their child's eating were more often reported by obese adults than by those of normal weight. The answer seems simple. Provide your child with a variety of healthy foods, and this doesn't just mean letting him choose crisps or chips, and allow him to choose what he wants. Revolutionary, maybe. But research over half a century would seem to back this up.

From all this research, one message still seems to come over loud and clear. The children did eat what they actually needed. If they did not need or want it, no one complained. In fact much of the worrying that parents do about their child's eating is a result of their expecting him to eat more than he needs. If a mother gives a four-year-old the same size portion as a ten-year-old, then she really should not be too surprised when he doesn't finish it.

One extremely useful way of seeing the problem more clearly is to keep a food diary for a few days. I well remember one mother who consulted me about her child's eating problem. 'He hardly eats a thing,' she told me. However, even while she was in my consulting room she was giving her son biscuits to keep him quiet. The child wasn't eating his meals because he was full from between-meal snacks. This is an extreme example, but lesser degrees are common. By keeping a detailed diary over a period of a few days in which you record absolutely everything that your child eats and drinks you may discover that he eats far more than you realized. I would recommend this approach to any parent whose children have any sort of feeding problem. However do not just keep a diary for one or two days. Children often go through phases of eating for a few days, and then stopping almost completely for a while. If you only record in one of these phases you will get a false picture. Make sure you take long enough to get a complete view of all his different eating phases, and then average them out. Most parents are surprised and relieved when they do this.

Remember that you are wasting your time, trying to force your child to eat something he doesn't like, and to eat a large portion when he wants only a little. If you really want to know how it feels give yourself a double size portion of everything at your next meal and ask your husband or wife to insist that you eat it up. You aren't allowed to leave the table until it has all gone. If you really want to see how many children experience feeding, then – when you really feel bloated – have your partner try and spoon more food into your mouth, pretending to be a train or aeroplane if necessary. Now put yourself in your child's shoes. How must it feel to a child to be treated like this? Is it any wonder they often spit food out when they have had enough? Wouldn't you have a temper tantrum too if it went on for long?

Your job as a provider of food for your child, purely from the nutritional point of view, is to offer a good selection of wholesome food in quantities the child wants to eat. If he only wants a teaspoonful, then give a teaspoonful. When he's hungry he'll ask for some more. I am well aware that your child cannot go through his entire life only eating what he wants when he wants. However, I am here simply laying down guidelines for those parents who are worried about their child's nutrition. We will return to discipline, and the social aspects of eating, later.

Could there be something wrong with him?

If a child who has always eaten well suddenly goes off his food it is important to find out why. Assuming there have been no changes in the sort of food you have offered, then there may well be some medical reason. These can be divided into two groups. There are conditions that make eating painful, and those that affect the appetite.

Painful conditions are usually easy to spot, provided you think about them. Teething, or any form of toothache, will make a child reluctant to eat solid foods. A sore mouth from gingivitis (inflammation of the gums), or tonsilitis or other forms of sore throat will also obviously make a child try to avoid eating and swallowing.

Loss of appetite is a very common symptom of a number of illnesses. All the virus illnesses, such as colds and flu, have this effect and should be reasonably obvious from the other symptoms. The list of possibilities is almost endless, and if your child has suddenly lost his appetite for no very good reason, and particularly if he seems unwell in any other way, do get your doctor to check him over.

What about the waste?

The old argument about insisting that your child should eat all his food because other children, especially in third world countries, are starving really makes no sense at all. If your child has eaten enough for his needs, then eating any more is just as much a waste as scraping it into the bin, or feeding it to the dog. Mothers often fall into the same trap. I regularly see overweight women who want to lose some of their extra pounds. When their dietary history is examined, they admit very frequently to finishing any food their children have left – particularly toast, cake, or chips – as 'it would be such a waste to throw it away'. How can eating food that you don't need, and which does nothing but make you overweight, be anything but a waste, too?

It makes infinitely more sense to offer children portions that they need, want, and will eat rather than portions that are too large and you have to nag them to finish. Unless you intend to parcel up the scraps on your child's plate and send them off to a starving third world family, then forget that argument. If you really want to help, have smaller meals and give the money you've saved to a suitable charity.

Discipline

The child of toddler age is a natural rebel. The psychologists call it 'toddler negativism', which is simply a way of saying that whatever you want a toddler to do, he won't. The toddler is trying to establish his place in the world, his role in the family. He likes to find out what will please you, and what will annoy you. Above all he likes a reaction. To get you into a furious mood all by himself may be seen as a great triumph. No longer is he an inactive part of the home. He is a major influence on how everyone thinks, feels and behaves – and he knows it.

Most feeding problems start at toddler age. The natural response to 'eat it up' is for the child to refuse. As a result, mealtimes become more and more tense as parents attempt to impose their will and children refuse. Discipline is, of course, tremendously important but there are better times than mealtimes to have your battles. As we have seen, food and feeding are very important to mothers, and if some of the reassuring principles of nutrition that I have discussed are not known, then the parents' anxiety level can rise and rise, creating just the effect the child wants.

Some parents have noticed their children are happier to eat ready-prepared commercial meals than home-cooked food. For the contrary toddler this may just be linked with his realizing how much more you care about his eating food you have slaved over, and feel hurt about when he doesn't eat it.

If you make mealtimes the occasion to have battles over discipline then I can guarantee two things. Mealtimes will be a misery, and your child will win. The less that mealtimes become battles, the more relaxed you will all be about feeding in general, and the more your child will begin to behave sociably at meals. If meals are fun, you can begin to have special 'grown-up' meals together – such as I suggested in Chapter 4 – and he will learn the social skills he needs for eating out, and at school.

I remember one mother who consulted me with a number of feeding worries. Her three-year-old daughter always wanted to eat her dessert before her main course was eaten. Invariably screaming and temper tantrums erupted on both sides.

I asked her why it was so important which order the foods were eaten in. Obviously from a nutritional point of view it cannot make any difference. However, she was worried that if she allowed this her child would still want to eat her courses the wrong way round when she started school. In other words, she was prepared to turn meal-times into something her daughter hated, for the sake of avoiding something that might never happen. A hatred of meals would be far more likely to cause problems than eating her meals back to front.

For two weeks she allowed her daughter to eat her dessert first. She would have let her go on for longer, but the child did not want to! Such problems can be as easy as that to solve. It is even easier not to see them as problems, but simply as your child finding out what his own mealtime preferences are. If you look at your differences of opinion in this way, then letting him experiment won't be seen in terms of you 'being weak' and 'letting him win'. The chances are you will all end up eating similar foods, but if he does like different things, then he has every right to. He may decide he doesn't like to eat much of the white of an egg. The rest of the family may enjoy it, and consider him faddy. But, what if he had been born into a family where no one liked egg whites? Would he have been labelled faddy then?

Many of the parents who wrote to me had tried every possible way of getting their child to eat, and had concluded that making a fuss was a waste of time. One mother who had learnt this lesson with her first child, after a great many battles, totally avoided all such arguments with the second. When this child was twenty months old, her mother wrote, 'So far Emily has never had any fads and has never refused to eat meals on a regular basis. I always treat her refusals as genuine dislike of a food and offer her an alternative. We have seen friends who shout at their children, as we used to, force them to eat, and do not allow a dessert if the first course is not finished. The children have always been faddy eaters who behave badly at table. Surely there is a link between our approach, and Emily's all-embracing appetite.'

Another mother wrote, 'My advice to parents is that if a child won't eat, *nothing* will make it, but don't worry – they won't let themselves starve.' Yet another revealed, 'I was much better when I stopped worrying, and when I closed my ears to other people's comments.'

How right these parents were. If you are reading this in the hope of avoiding feeding problems, then you will be more aware of that attitude to take. However, if you have read this far because your child has problems now, and you want specific advice, try and remember the following:

- Decide what you are worried about.

  After reading the earlier part of this chapter you may realize that your worry is unnecessary, particularly when you remember how little harm will come to your child. Given a free choice of good foods, he won't starve.
- Remember – it takes two to make a quarrel.
- Serve less than your child will eat – not more.

  It is far better to give your child more of a particular food later, if he asks, than to overface him from the start. Let your child say how much he wants. If you eat at a restaurant that is what you tell the waiter. Isn't it reasonable to treat your child the same way?
- Don't rush your child.

  If he is taking a long time to finish, then leave him to do so. The rest of you can get on with the next course, or other activities. Hurrying will lead to tension, and you know what that does.
- Don't nag your child.

  Don't be surprised if your child doesn't want to eat if you've spent the mealtime coaxing, nagging, threatening and criticizing. Anxiety makes the stomach feel all knotted up, hardly guaranteed to help the appetite. Wait till after the meal if you want to comment on table manners, school reports, and so on.
- Keep a food diary.

  This will not only reveal exactly how much your child does eat, which may put your mind at rest, but should show when he is hungry and when there are problems. With this information you can . . .

- Think about the timing of meals.

   Are you making your child wait too long for a meal, or feeding him too often or too soon after the previous meal? A common problem is the child who is made to wait until the rest of the family have arrived home from work before he has his evening meal. The child may be both too hungry, and overtired – not a recipe for a happy meal.
- Try to keep his meals to a regular routine, whenever possible.
- Don't worry about finger feeding.

   As long as your child can master a knife and fork by the time he goes to school, then don't worry if he uses his fingers at two or three years old. He will soon want to imitate the grown-ups, but finger feeding at least makes sure some food gets in.
- Make food look fun to eat.

   The reluctant eater will be more tempted by colourful dips and attractive meals than by dollops of dull-looking mush.
- Don't worry about his strange tastes.

   If he will only eat potatoes if they are smothered in tomato sauce, he won't come to harm. If you refuse to let him dip bread in his custard, he may refuse to eat either. It is much better to look the other way.
- Don't worry about the order of courses.

   If he insists on having dessert first, then let him. He will insist more and more if you refuse. No one will have any peace and the meal will be a misery. If you allow it, he will soon change to the more conventional approach.
- Try and involve him in food preparation.

   From the age of three your child can help with simple tasks in preparing a meal or snack. The child who never drinks milk may happily drink a glass full if allowed to mix a milk shake. Even being allowed to help wash fruit or vegetables may stimulate some interest in eating them.

● Don't serve food that you know he doesn't like.

Forcing a child to eat a food will never make him like it. Far better to give the child something different (and simple to make) if the rest of the family is having something he doesn't relish. Sooner or later he may well ask to try a bit.

● Your child must be reasonable too.

It is not acceptable for him to have all of a particular dish if the rest of the family wants some too. He can have his fair share, but not more. Favourite areas for arguments like this include the crackling on meat, the skin on rice pudding, and the top of apple crumbles!

● Don't use bribes.

Offering the child an extra treat if he eats a food he doesn't want rarely succeeds – for long. Parents try gold stars, sweets, or even extra pocket money. It may work once or twice, but you can be certain that it won't last. The child will expect the stakes to be raised. In addition, yet again bribery like this makes eating seem a chore to be endured, not a pleasure to be enjoyed.

● Watch the drinks.

Many children who seem to have small appetites have problems because they drink so much at a mealtime. If a four- or five-year-old drinks a glassful of lemon or orange squash at the beginning of a meal, then it really is not surprising if there is not much room left for the rest.

● Don't insist on 'just one mouthful'.

There is nothing to be gained from insisting that

your child tries a food he is reluctant to taste. You are likely to make him even more determined that he won't eat it and won't enjoy it.

- Make life easier for yourself.

It is well worth getting your child used to eating foods that are easy for you to prepare, and are likely to be available wherever you go. A child who will eat cheese is marvellously easy to cater for, whether you are at home or abroad. If he will have biscuits or fruit as well you have the makings of a perfectly satisfactory meal.

- Ignore other people's children.

An important study performed as long ago as 1947 by the Medical Research Council looked at the diets of over a thousand children. This showed huge variations in their intake of Calories. Some children consumed twice as many Calories as others while remaining similar in size and growth rate. The author of this study concluded: 'Individual requirements must differ as much as individual intakes, and that an average intake, however valuable statistically, should never be used to assess an individual's requirements.' In other words, if your friends' children seem to eat far more or far less than your own child it is only interesting, not worrying.

Above all . . .

- Make mealtimes fun. The less you all argue and shout at each other, the less there will be to argue and shout about. Try it and see.

6

Snacks and Sweets

'My husband and I both decided when she was a young baby that we were going to stick to certain rules when it came to snacks. She could have fruit. She could have milk or water. Anything else and we were going to put our foot down. We didn't want one of those children who is always chewing sweets or crisps! It didn't turn out that way. We felt so cruel when her friends came to play that we had to give in. It was hopeless.'

More parents have good intentions about between-meals-eating than almost any other aspect of nutrition. Snacks seem so unnecessary, and the foods that children choose seem so awful, that many parents become quite determined that their child won't be like 'all the others'. They are rarely successful. There are so many other pressures on children to ask for snacks that parental intentions often get swept away.

Of all the reasons that children demand food between meals, hunger is perhaps the most acceptable one. In addition habit, boredom, parental pressure, and advertising all play a part. Hunger is often understandable. Most children get peckish in the mid-mornings, and also after school or halfway through the afternoon. This particularly applies to the child who has eaten poorly at breakfast or the midday meal, but having a large snack at this time of the day may result in the child not feeling hungry at the next meal and a vicious circle gets established. Snacking takes away hunger, which means a small meal is taken, which leads to hunger a few hours later, which leads to another snack – and so on, ad infinitum. I have certainly come across many children who eat more between meals than they do at mealtimes. In the last chapter I mentioned the mother who consulted me about her five-yearold son who apparently 'never ate a thing'. In fact he munched a packet of biscuits in my consulting room as his mother unfolded her series of worries. She had given him the biscuits to 'keep him quiet', and did not seem to realize either that they were food, or that they were bound to dull his appetite for the next meal.

Parents frequently give snacks as rewards, or as a simple way of keeping a bored child quiet. Boredom is a very potent cause of snacking. The child who is busy with a model or puzzle is far less likely to demand something to eat than the child who is sitting about watching television. Indeed research at Cornell University in the USA has shown that the more television children watch the more sweet foods they eat. Specifically, for every two hours of television watched, children ate another sweet such as cake, candy, biscuits, or ice-cream. They suggested that this might be linked to exposure to advertising, though inactivity and boredom may well be important too. This same research also showed that other factors influenced sweet consumption, in particular the amount of sweets that parents consume, and also the parents' attitudes towards sweets. Children of parents who had 'positive attitudes' towards sweets – those most likely to use sweets as rewards or treats – ate three times as many sweets per day as children whose parents discouraged sweet-eating.

Why should snack and sweet-eating be a problem?

After all, in the last chapter I looked at meals in general and concluded that there is no right or wrong way to structure your day's eating. Nothing except convention dictates that food must be eaten in main meals with no snacks in between.

No, the problems do not relate to the existence or timing of snacks, but more to the quality of what is eaten and its effect on what else is eaten during the rest of the day. A child who eats reasonably sized meals of good food, and has regular or occasional nutritious snacks, does not have a problem. The child who is constantly eating junk food between meals to the exclusion of a reasonably healthy mixed diet at mealtimes may certainly cause concern.

The most common items to be eaten between meals are processed foods, particularly those containing refined and processed carbohydrates, french fries – or chips, as we used to call them! – and sweets. All of these have their own particular problems, and most of them are extensively and expensively marketed. Healthier substitutes, such as fresh fruit, rarely get the television advertising specifically aimed at children that chocolate bars and bags of potato-based snacks receive.

Perhaps sweets and chocolates are the biggest villains. Sugar is still eaten in vast quantities, with the average American and Briton eating a hundred pounds of sugar every year. In Chapter 1 I discussed some of the ways in which sugar can be 'hidden' in your food, but it is worth remembering that sugar may not be labelled simply as 'sugar' on packaging. There are in fact two main types of sugar – the monosaccharides, composed of single molecules, and the disaccharides, with double molecules. They all have names ending in '-ose'. Sucrose is the most widely used sugar and is made up of equal parts of glucose and fructose. White table sugar is nothing other than sucrose. Nowadays one often sees products marketed as containing fructose or glucose, as if one type was better for you than another. This isn't the case. Similarly brown sugar is simply sucrose coloured with molasses, and unrefined raw sugar is no more nourishing for you than white sugar. Alas, the advantages of sweetening with honey are so small as to be insignificant, despite the claims of honey enthusiasts. I am not decrying honey's splendid taste, just any claims for real nutritional superiority.

Perhaps the best-known sugar-related problem is tooth decay, and research has shown that sweets eaten with meals are far less damaging to teeth than those eaten between meals. It is possible that other foods counter some of sugar's harmful effects on teeth. Unfortunately the trend in recent years has been away from the sweet, or dessert, at the end of a meal and more to the between-meal snack. From the point of view of your children's teeth, it is far better to allow them sweets at a mealtime, and better still if they brush their teeth after the meal.

The other great problem with sugar is the effect on weight. While sugar itself is not particularly fattening, sweets are a very concentrated way of taking Calories. Your child can munch large quantities of them before he begins to feel full. On the other hand, if he eats fruit or bread he will feel full very quickly. A couple of bananas is likely to fill any child, but contains far fewer Calories than a single chocolate wafer biscuit that may well leave him feeling hungry. In other words, eating the snack as fruit would fill him using fewer Calories than eating the snack as chocolate or sweets. Not only that, but the fruit will provide fibre and vitamins, definitely absent from sweets.

Many adults seem to have a form of addiction to sugar, needing their daily fix of sweets or chocolate. Such a sweet tooth invariably results from the habits of childhood. Incidentally, you can ignore those advertising claims for sugar as being a source of instant energy. In fact the opposite is often true. A concentrated dose of sugar 'fools' the body into thinking more food is likely to follow. The body's production of insulin is rapidly increased so that there will be enough to deal with the whole meal. When the meal doesn't arrive, the extra insulin inevitably clears too much sugar from the blood and you can end up feeling even more tired and hungry than before the snack. Higher fibre snacks have no such negative side-effects.

Another very popular type of snack is based around potatoes. French fries, or chips, are a particular favourite away from home, while crisps and other semi-synthetic substitutes in all manner of extraordinary shapes and flavours – including smoky bacon flavoured space-ships – are tremendously popular as nibbles during TV programmes. Dentists are far happier with these sorts of foods than they are with sweets, but other health care professionals are far less keen. The director of the blood pressure unit at London's Charing Cross Hospital has even gone so far as to say, 'If we got nutritionalists to devise the worst possible diet for the development of cardiovascular disease, that is what we are giving our children today. The seeds of heart disease and high blood pressure start in early childhood.'

He is referring to the salt content of such snacks. A high salt intake is an important factor in the development of high blood pressure, and the early habit of eating salty snacks makes the tastebuds less sensitive to salt. As a result more is sprinkled on to food at mealtimes to make it seem less bland. It may seem absurd to worry about your child having a stroke or heart attack later in life as a result of developing a liking for salt now, but the evidence all points to this as being the case.

On a more optimistic note, one splendid trend in the UK over recent years has been the increased availability of baked potatoes as a hot snack. In my wife's home town the market place has a chip shop at the entrance where the tempting smell of frying chips can be nearly irresistible on a cold winter's afternoon. Just a few yards further on an equally delicious smell drifts through the air from a small baked potato stand which has recently appeared. Happily there is far less reason to resist its temptation!

A medium-sized baked potato has about 115 Calories, and a small pat of butter or margarine adds just over 30 Calories although a good potato can be tasty enough on its own. The Consumer's Union in the USA has shown that a baked potato in its skin rivals beans in nutritional value and beats noodles, rice, or white bread.

If you decide to eat the same potato in the form of french fries, however, you will instead take in the grand total of 420 Calories. Potato crisps are equally bad. An ounce of potato crisps contains 151 Calories (133 Calories per 25 grams). There seems little doubt that the baked potato makes a nutritionally more sensible purchase.

However, the news on potato crisps is not all bad. At least one major UK crisp producer now claims to use a high proportion of polyunsaturated cooking oil, mainly consisting of soyabean oil or rapeseed oil as blends with palm oil or on their own. In addition I have noticed the following wording appear on the package of one of the UK's most popular potato crisps: 'They make a useful contribution to dietary fibre and have no added sucrose.' If nothing else this shows how much more aware consumers are becoming about dietary matters. Nevertheless, it seemed a little vague in its claims. The company concerned told me they did not quote figures on the pack as there had been no national decision as to how fibre content should be standardized, but in general the fibre content of crisps is quoted as 11.9 gm per 100 gm. An average pack therefore contains around 3 gm of fibre. Current recommendations for adults aim at an intake of 30 gm per day.

Biscuits have many of the same disadvantages as sweets. They are high in Calories, and low in nutritional value. The occasional biscuit will do no harm, but do not leave your child to help himself from the biscuit tin. Few children know when to stop, and before you know where you are they will be too full to eat their next meal.

So, what policy should you take over sweets and snacks? The simplest answer would be to ban them completely. Indeed this sort of advice used to be commonplace. In Mabel Liddiard's *The Mothercraft Manual* published in 1928 is the comment, 'Allow no sweets or scraps between meals . . . a fairy story with a greedy fairy and sad results is the best illustration.' Would that life were that simple. For many children some form of snack is important. The small size of a child's stomach may not be adequate to take in enough food at a meal to last them through the five hours to the next meal. Indeed few young children manage to consume enough Calories in three set meals to meet their daily needs.

Unquestionably friends will eat snacks and sweets, even if you ban them, and to single your child out may seem extremely harsh. The problem is compounded by the fact that even four-year-olds are quite able to help themselves to biscuits and similar snacks and a ban for the child, and not yourself, would entail locking the doors of food cupboards. Is that what you really want? Instead, may I offer the following suggestions:

- Don't buy foods that you don't want your children to eat. You can hardly be surprised if they clamour for foods that they know are sitting there in the cupboard. It may seem ridiculously simple advice, but many parents find it much easier to say 'No, I haven't got' than 'No, you can't have'.

- Restrict eating to certain rooms in the house – usually the kitchen and dining-room. The child who sits in front of the television with a plate of snacks is likely to eat far more than he really wants or needs.

- Be tough in the supermarket. Food retailers are not stupid. They position tempting snacks at child height near the checkout, where tempers are often getting frayed and parents are likely to buy anything to keep their nagging children quiet. Once you have given in, your children are even more likely to nag next time. It is worth giving them some sort of acceptable pacifier before you get to the sweet counter, or if it is possible, shop alone.

- Instead of sweets, make sure you keep plenty of fresh fruit, nuts, and raisins in the house.

- Don't use sweets as a reward. In particular avoid the temptation to say at a mealtime that if your child eats all his meat then he can have a sweet later. Just think of the impression of the two different foodstuffs that sort of comment gives your child.

- Beware of advertisements. With older children you can make a game out of spotting how the sweet and snack advertisers present their biased messages. Get them to ask questions about the adverts such as the pertinent question 'than what' about the claim 'now even more nourishing'.

- Instead of buying cakes and sweets try making your own. It is obviously more time-consuming, but at least you will know what your child is eating. There are many healthy recipes around nowadays, and on standard recipes you can always improve things by reducing the sugar content by up to a third.

- Be sceptical about some of the apparently healthy

89

snack bars now coming on to the market. Increasing awareness of nutritional problems has made this a growth area, and while some are excellent, others are no better than conventional candy bars, despite the 'natural and wholesome' claims on the wrappers.

- Avoid getting into the habit of always giving sweets at the same time each day, for instance, after school. Try and ring the changes with the snacks. Some families restrict sweets to a once-weekly treat, often after a particular meal. The child may see this as more of a treat than unlimited sweets the rest of the time.
- Pocket money poses problems. You can either let your child choose how to spend his money himself – which obviously he has to eventually – but risk his spending it all on sweets, or else give a separate sweet allowance which you yourself choose and distribute. Neither method is perfect, but if you've followed the other suggestions your child is unlikely to have developed a sweet tooth and may prefer to buy books, comics or toys instead.
- Finally, beware nagging too much at mealtimes. Constantly telling your child to 'eat it up' will make him tense and anxious and anxiety lessens the appetite, making him even less likely to finish his food. Once the meal is over, the anxiety goes and the appetite returns. The demand for snacks between meals may sometimes be the result of mealtime nagging, rather than the snacks being the cause of the poor mealtime appetite. Make mealtimes a pleasure!

The Underweight Child

*'I really don't know what to do with her. She seems
to eat all right but she's just skin and bone. Should
I be feeding her extra Calories, or is it vitamins, or
what?'*

Though underweight children are far, far rarer than fat
children, and by far the commonest nutritional problem
in affluent societies is obesity, nevertheless parents are far
more likely to worry if their child looks thin than if he
looks chubby.

It is all too easy to be mistaken if you simply judge a
child by how he looks. Even a perfectly healthy, fit, and
athletic child may have ribs that stick out, a protruding
belly, and seemingly non-existent muscles. Parents can
get all too easily confused if they start worrying about how
their child looks in the bath.

The absolutely essential thing to do if you suspect your
child might be at all underweight is to keep a growth
chart. I have already explained the principles behind such
charts at some length in Chapter 3. You will recall that
this is a simple way of comparing your child's actual
growth with his expected growth. By taking even a single
reading of your child's weight and height you will have
some idea of how he compares with other children of the
same age. However, it is even more valuable to plot

several such readings on the graph to gauge if he is growing at the rate one would expect. Don't forget that a single measurement of weight cannot tell you if he is putting on weight faster than he should, less than he should, or is just right.

The vast majority of parents who are worried about their children being underweight will be reassured, and often surprised, by the charts. Nevertheless for a small group of children underweight and small size remain serious and significant problems.

It is first worth considering the child who is both short and underweight, or even just short. By definition, three out of a hundred children will be below the third percentile on the growth charts. Unfortunately, children being the sort of creatures they are, this may well prove to be a source of considerable unhappiness for them. Teasing of short children is all too common, and while some small children will admit to being upset and embarrassed, others will bear the teasing silently, and may become excessively shy, aggressive and withdrawn.

Having accurately recorded your child's height and finding that he is below the third percentile, it would be wise to repeat the measurement after three months and then to take these recordings, and any earlier ones, along to your doctor for him to assess the next course of action.

Your doctor will then be able to put your child in one of four groups, and will act accordingly. If your child is unwell in any way, and if his growth rate has actually shown signs of slowing down, then the doctor will almost certainly wish to arrange further investigations, probably by referral to hospital. I will return to this group shortly.

The doctor may decide your child is short for genetic reasons. If either parent is short, then obviously this is likely to mean the child is short, and one way that this cause can be established is by working out what is called the 'mid-parental centile'. This adjusts the chart to be more specifically accurate for your child, by shifting the fiftieth centile to the position of your child's expected height.

This isn't as complicated as it sounds. In order to calculate a boy's expected height you plot the father's height on the centile chart, and the mother's height plus 12.5 cm (5 in). The midpoint between these is the boy's eventual expected height – in other words the new fiftieth centile for that child. For a girl, the mother's height is plotted, and the father's height minus 12.5 cm (5 in) and the midpoint between these is the girl's expected height. When these adjustments have been made it may well become apparent that growth is perfectly satisfactory for that child in that family.

Social deprivation is another potent cause of failure to thrive by a child, and is often associated with poor health and malnutrition. Obviously a doctor will want to make arrangements for appropriate treatment and care of such a child.

Finally the doctor may decide that the child is probably nothing more than a late developer and simply needs observation and measurement after a year. This group typically includes the child who is perfectly fit, but whose height falls to a point below the normal range after school entry, and particularly after the age of ten. This sort of child is usually, but not always, developing more slowly than his colleagues and as the growth chart reflects the average for his age he will temporarily appear to have fallen behind.

Of the group that require hospital assessment there are obviously many possible causes that need to be excluded. One of the most important, and which affects about one in four thousand children, is growth hormone deficiency (GHD). Growth hormone is a hormone that is normally produced by the pituitary gland, situated at the base of the brain, and a baby born with this condition will not grow as normally expected. The condition can occasionally develop later in children who have had radiotherapy to the head for treatment of cancer. Growth hormone deficiency, if detected early, is totally treatable. Without treatment a boy with this condition is unlikely to grow to more than 4 ft 6 in, and a girl to 4 ft 2 in. If treatment is started by the age of two or three years, then the child will reach a perfectly normal height. If treatment is delayed until the age of five or six, then boys will reach 5 ft 4 in, and girls 4 ft 11 in. You can see the importance of early detection and treatment! However at present the average age of referral to a specialist is between eight and nine. Wider use of growth charts is very obviously urgently needed.

When the diagnosis is confirmed, treatment consists of injections of growth hormone and many units encourage parents to give the injections themselves, a small price to pay for normal growth. During such treatment, which may continue until after adolescence when normal growth ceases, your child will be regularly measured and tested. Currently the growth hormone used for treatment is a synthetic hormone produced by DNA technology. Brands include Genotropin, Humatrope, and Norditropin, which are identical in structure to the natural hormone, and inevitably extremely expensive – but worth every penny.

Other vitally important conditions have to be looked for and either excluded or treated. A medical text book is really the place to list the numerous causes, many of which are extremely rare, and I cannot possibly deal with them all here. Clearly the child's nutrition and general health will need to be fully assessed. As a rule, a child who is short and overweight is likely to have a glandular, hormonal, problem. A child who is short and underweight may have almost anything wrong and needs full detailed assessment.

Two particular causes are well worth mentioning briefly, however. Coeliac disease is diagnosed in about one person in fifteen hundred in the UK, though there is wide national variation and in parts of Western Ireland it affects one in three hundred.

In this condition the lining of the bowel is affected by gluten – a protein that is present in wheat, rye, barley and oats which makes it lose its fluffy texture and become smooth. Being smooth it is much less able to absorb nutrients. As a result the children fail to thrive and tend to develop diarrhoea. By leaving gluten completely out of the diet the lining of the bowel fully recovers and the child then grows completely normally. The diet must be continued for the rest of the sufferer's life. If this condition is diagnosed in your child, I would very strongly recommend that you join the Coeliac Society. The address is given at the end of the book.

The other condition affecting growth that many people have heard of is cystic fibrosis, in which the pancreas fails to produce enzymes which normally digest proteins, carbohydrates and fats and allow them to be absorbed. Much of the goodness in the food therefore passes straight through the body. The condition also affects the lining of the lungs, and afflicted children tend to have numerous respiratory infections and coughs. The condition affects about one in every two thousand babies born, and tends to run in families. If it runs in your family, and you are considering having a child, do ask your doctor to refer you to a genetic counsellor.

The treatment of cystic fibrosis involves giving extracts of animal pancreas in powder form. In the past the amount of fat in the diet was reduced, but nowadays this is far less important with adequate use of the enzyme supplements.

Obviously the respiratory infections also require special treatment, including regular physiotherapy. Again there is a useful group for parents and sufferers, and the address is at the end of the book.

Don't forget, these conditions are generally very rare, and yet three in a hundred children are below the third centile for height and weight. If your child is in this group the chances are still high that he will be fine, but it is essential that you get him checked over.

If your child does not have any of these specific conditions, is a normal height, but seems underweight and skinny, then his problems obviously should not be ignored. First of all you must determine whether he is actually suffering at all from his thinness. Is he being teased, or doesn't it bother him half as much as it bothers you? You must be sure you know why you are concerned. It is important that children come to accept themselves as they truly are, and don't think of themselves as being inferior. The weakling in the old Charles Atlas advertisments had sand kicked in his face more because of his attitude to himself and the world than because of his actual size.

If your child seems to eat well, then it is well worth keeping a detailed diary of what he eats over a period of a week. In this he should record absolutely everything that he eats and drinks. Check up on the amount of protein that he eats, and also the total Calories intake. You may see obvious areas for improvement, but don't forget – no amount of extra Calories and vitamins can turn your child into something that genetically he was not destined to be. If he is destined to be 5 ft tall, extra food can only make him fatter, not a six-footer.

I have deliberately left the topic of anorexia nervosa to the end of this chapter. Many parents think of this topic when they are worried that their child is too thin. In the past it was thought that it was only a disease of adolescents, with young children not being at risk. Sadly, this is certainly no longer the case, although it is still rare in the young child. Unfortunately it is also possible that it is under-diagnosed, because many general practitioners and even paediatricians fail to take it into account as even a possibility, mistakenly believing that it does not occur at a young age.

The condition is, however, almost entirely different to the type of food refusal that affects the average young child. It is characterized by an overwhelming refusal to eat that can lead to an extreme loss of weight. This may well be associated with disturbances in the body's hormones, and occasionally may even lead to death. It is about fifteen times commoner in girls than boys, and its incidence has increased considerably in recent years. Certain groups are more at risk than others. For example a study of schoolgirls in England aged sixteen or over in 1976 showed an incidence of 1 in 250, while in Canada a study of ballet students in 1978 showed 6 per cent were sufferers. The condition is commoner among the upper social classes, but no social class is completely immune.

The cause of the condition is something of a mystery. It is neither entirely a physical condition nor entirely a psychological condition. On a very simple level it can be seen as a fear of getting fat. A sensitive teenager may be teased by her friends, or overhear someone saying that she is fat. This can set her off on a strict diet, which then gets out of control. However, as the huge majority of teenagers who try to lose weight do not go on to get the condition, this simplistic theory is insufficient. Some of the sufferers appear subconsciously to dread the prospect of growing up, of sexual feelings, or of leaving home. Remaining very thin seems to help avoid these possibilities. If the breasts become very small, for example, an obvious element in the girl's sexuality is affected. Such problems seem more likely if there are tensions in the family, particularly some form of marital disharmony.

However, such psychological causes are not the whole answer as in some female patients it has been recorded that their periods stop before they begin to lose weight. Whenever it occurs, the cessation of periods (amenorrhoea) is almost universal among female sufferers. In boys the chief hormonal change is a loss of sexual interest and potency. It is still hotly debated as to whether such hormonal changes are cause or effect.

Whatever the cause, the picture of the illness is fairly standard. Typically occurring in girls aged fourteen to seventeen, the sufferer initially begins to follow a slimming diet, frequently cutting down dramatically on carbohydrates, and often begins to exercise far more. At first all this may appear to be a very healthy development. However, as the condition goes on the weight loss becomes a preoccupation. The sufferer becomes genuinely convinced that he or she is still fat, and the perception of his or her own body image is grossly distorted. To anyone else the girl may appear very slim, but to herself she still appears plump. Occasionally people with this condition make themselves vomit after eating. This is particularly common if they have just been on a binge of over-eating; a curious but not infrequent occurrence. Laxatives may also be grossly overused in an attempt to stop food being absorbed.

Actual nutritional problems are remarkably few. Fat is the chief tissue to be lost from the body. Protein is relatively well-preserved, and vitamin deficiencies are surprisingly uncommon. The chief problems are psychological, rather than physical, and the 5 per cent fatality rate from the condition is mainly due to suicide. Depression is very common and needs careful and expert treatment.

The chief aims in treating the condition are to obtain the sufferer's confidence and co-operation (often an exceedingly difficult matter), to restore her weight to its previous healthy level, and to shorten the length of the illness. The majority of sufferers require in-patient treatment at a suitable psychiatric unit. As well as close supervision of eating, psychotherapy may help unravel the causes and gently encourage the patient to return to a normal life style. This may take a great deal of time, and any psychological, sexual, or domestic conflicts will need exploring.

The course of anorexia nervosa is variable, but frequently lasts two or three years. Relapses may occur but about 70 per cent make a complete recovey. Anorexia nervosa is a complex condition, and is covered in considerably more detail in my book, *Bulimia: A guide for sufferers and their families*, also published by Cedar Paperbacks. This book also looks at the other forms of eating disorder which are sadly becoming so much commoner in young adults.

Obesity

'My husband and I are both overweight, so I suppose we shouldn't be surprised that Joanne is as well. Her friends are beginning to tease her dreadfully, but I don't want to make her neurotic by making her go on a strict diet. It doesn't seem fair at her age.'

You only have to go into any newsagent's shop to see evidence of the huge interest there is in being slim. Row after row of magazines are devoted to losing weight, all of them full of advertisements for foods or other devices that are supposed to help you 'shed those unwanted pounds'. Slimness is the fashion. Slim is successful. A study of body types portrayed on television even showed that fewer than one in fifty of the actors were significantly overweight.

However, it is only a fashion. You only have to look at the paintings of Rubens. The women pictured so voluptuously are hardly the waif-like supermodels of the 1990s. Indeed, they are distinctly plump. Look at the paintings by Titian, or Renoir. The women those chose to glorify in their paintings would never have had the slightest chance of being shortlisted for a job in modelling in our culture.

Quite simply, different cultures at different times find different physical attributes attractive. Indeed, it has been estimated that eight out of ten of the world's cultures consider a degree of overweight to be desirable for women, and in nine out of ten cultures fat thighs are deemed attractive.

However, there really is more to the question of obesity than simply worrying about fashion. Minor degrees of overweight really do not matter, but the genuinely fat do have more illnesses. Fat adults are far more likely to develop coronary artery disease, with the subsequent risk of heart attacks. There is also an increased risk of developing diabetes, gallstones, osteoarthritis, and having complications after any form of surgery. For a man who is 60 per cent overweight, the chance of an early death is twice that of someone of average weight at the same height. For women the risk is two-thirds greater.

Most of these problems are fairly easy to understand. For instance, if the body is larger than it was intended to be, is it any wonder that the extra strain on the hip joints causes arthritis and pain? However, other effects of obesity take more explaining. The obese teenager is only half as likely to be admitted to college as his slim colleague, even with the same academic qualifications. Indeed, a fat business executive is in general paid less, and less likely to be promoted, than a thin one.

It is clear that society really does put a premium on slimness. Everyone is bombarded with the message that slim is beautiful. If you want to be sexy, fit, popular, happy, and successful then you have to be slim. And if you are overweight then you are probably lazy, unable to control yourself – in short, a slob.

Such prejudices are not unique to adults, but are learnt at a very early age. An interesting study in America asked children to look at a series of six drawings of children. One was 'normal', one had a brace on one leg and used crutches, one was in a wheelchair, one lacked a hand, one had a significantly disfigured face, and one was fat. The children in the study were asked to rank these in order of likeability. The least liked child of all was almost always the fat child.

There can be little doubt that when it comes to obesity, then prevention really is always better than cure, and if being careful about your child's weight can save a lifetime of dieting, then the problem of childhood obesity is well worth detailed consideration – particularly when most adult diets are so unsuccessful. Depressingly, it has been calculated that around 85 per cent of all weight lost on diets is subsequently regained.

It is important to be clear exactly what is meant by obesity – a word that comes from the Latin *obesus*, meaning 'fat, stout, plump, or stupid', an interesting definition. Sometimes the condition is all too apparent. One of the heaviest women on record was Flora Jackson. She was a big baby who became an obese child, an obese adult, and then died young. At birth she weighed 4.5 kg (9 lb 14 oz), 121 kg (19 stone) at eleven years and 381 kg (60 stone) when she died at the age of thirty-five.

For most children and adults the definition is less clear-cut. Strictly speaking, a child is obese if his weight is more than 20 per cent above the predicted weight for his height and sex. You will have to use the charts in Chapter 3 and your pocket calculator to work that one out. Doctors also assess obesity by measuring the thickness of skin folds in certain parts of the body, such as the upper arm or over the shoulder blade. In practice, however, you can almost always be certain that if a child looks overweight, he is overweight. Indeed, one of the best definitions of childhood obesity that I have seen is 'a child who is too fat for his or her own good.' Using the charts will give you some guidance on this. Even if your child seems only a little too fat, the advice in this chapter is still worth reading. It would be absurd to wait until fatness reaches an arbitrarily agreed point before deciding that action needs taking. It cannot be said often enough. Preventing obesity is not only better than cure, it is much easier than cure.

Childhood obesity is very common; indeed it is the most prevalent and serious nutritional disease of childhood in both the USA and UK. Detailed estimates vary, but a study of Boston school children showed 10 per cent were significantly overweight. In the United Kingdom, when twelve thousand Leicester school children were examined in 1965, 303 were found to be 'grossly overweight'. (Interestingly, over 80 per cent of these came from lower income group families.)

Why should we be concerned about fat children? It is clear that fat adults have numerous problems, but is the same true of children? Indeed, are fat children more likely to become fat adults?

Unquestionably the health of fat children does suffer. Simple problems such as shortness of breath on exertion are fairly common. After all, a six-year-old who is 10 lb overweight is carrying a load equivalent to twenty packs of butter, or five bags of sugar, around with him. Little wonder that this extra strain has an effect. The extremely fat child can even develop a form of heart failure, and obesity is the leading cause of raised blood pressure in childhood. Emotional problems are also very common, but I will return to these later. In general serious physical problems are rare, and nowhere near as important as they are with fat adults.

The question of whether fat children become fat adults is harder to settle, but the answer is almost certainly a qualified 'yes'. It was shown several years ago that excess weight gain as early as six weeks old is strongly correlated with obesity at six to eight years of age. Another study has shown that if a child's weight hits the ninetieth percentile on the growth charts discussed in Chapter 3 at least once in the first six months of life, then that person is over two and a half times more likely to be overweight at the age of twenty. Of course, this does mean that some children can be significantly overweight and yet be normal as adults, so please don't despair that if your child is fat then he is doomed to remain so. However the risks are higher, so it is worth taking note.

The most important factors that determine what will happen to the fat child are the age of onset and the severity. It has been clearly shown that the incidence of obesity is pretty constant throughout childhood and adolescence, except for a slightly increased risk with teenage girls. The later the child has the problem, the less likely he is to recover.

About eight out of ten obese adolescents will become obese adults. About a third of adults who are obese will have been obese during childhood, but of the very obese adults the chance is nearer three-quarters. It seems that childhood obesity does account for a disproportionately large share of grossly obese adults – another reason to be careful.

The degree of obesity is also a measure of how likely the condition is to improve. It will come as no surprise that researchers have shown that the greater the severity of the obesity, the less likely it is to disappear spontaneously. Incidentally, obese children are more likely to go through puberty a year or so earlier than their school friends. However their final height will be only average, as growth also seems to slow and stop earlier.

Any consideration of what can be done about childhood obesity must look at why the problem occurs. If you have one obese child, there is a considerable risk that any future children will be fat too, so understanding the possible causes may help you prevent problems.

In general, obesity is due to an imbalance between the amount of energy taken in as food, and the amount of energy the child or adult uses up. Unfortunately, it is not quite as simple as that, as genetic factors do complicate the picture considerably – and even they are not straightforward.

From the start it is worth saying that 'gland problems' are actually very rare. For years 'it's his glands' has been an acceptable excuse for obesity, but it is an excuse that really should not be used. There are a number of rare medical causes of obesity, often with magnificent names such as adipososkeletogenitodystrophy, but in almost all of these the child is short as well as being fat. If the growth charts do show that your child is significantly short for his age, then you should get him checked over by your doctor. If not, a hormonal or glandular cause is most unlikely.

To consider the various possible causes of obesity, I will look at the intake and output sides of the energy balance separately. Too much intake is, of course, by far the commonest cause, and it frequently starts very early in life because fat babies are still regarded as 'bonny'. Chubby thighs are seen as evidence that a child is developing and growing well. This would be an understandable cause of pride for parents in countries where starvation is common, and where such fat could be seen as 'money in the bank', but it should afford no pleasure in the average Western family.

Early plumpness results from parents giving too much food. Introducing solids too early is perhaps the commonest reason. It is unnecessary to introduce solids before an infant is about four months of age; the usual mistake made is that because a young baby is crying then he must be hungry and dissatisfied with the feeds he has had. There are many other causes of crying – ranging from boredom and loneliness to discomfort or pain. Please don't feel you have to start offering cereals to the six-week-old baby, just because he is crying. You will end up with a fat baby, but not necessarily a happier one.

The other danger to young infants happens with bottle-fed babies whose parents put more than the instructed amount of powder in the bottle. This extra-concentrated milk can be dangerous, actually making the baby more thirsty. The thirst may make him cry, and this crying may be misinterpreted as hunger – and yet more milk gets given.

In general breast-fed babies are less likely to be obese than bottle-fed. I suspect that this has little to do with the quality of the milk. Bottle-fed babies are frequently fed until all the milk in the bottle has gone. Sometimes this even means jiggling the child to prevent him from sleeping until the last few drops are finished. This over-feeding is a habit that may be one of the major causes of obesity throughout our lives. How many of us stop eating when we are full? We usually eat till our plate is clean, whether we need the food or not. You can see why this causes problems when you realize that – for an adult – eating only an extra half slice of bread each day, over and above what is needed by the body, adds up to a grand total of 11,000 Calories a year. The habit of expecting our children to finish every mouthful of food or drink that we present to them may be a very potent cause of long-term obesity, and it probably starts with the encouragement to finish the bottle. Breast-fed babies are spared this extra food. They stop feeding when they are full, and as breasts are thankfully not yet fitted with meters to measure milk production, mothers do not feel obliged to get them to take any more.

The importance of the amount of food a child eats was shown extremely clearly in an American study in which four families were observed where there was an obese and nonobese brother within two years of the same age. In all four families the obese boys ate far more than their nonobese brothers at dinner (766 against 504 Calories) and the mothers served their obese sons far more food. The more slender boys left more food on their plate, and took much longer over their meals. There were far fewer differences between the two groups when it came to exercise outside the home, though the obese boys were much less active inside the home.

There is no doubt that with the older child overeating is by far the most important cause of fatness. This may happen because a child helps himself to large quantities of snacks, or it may be because parents are constantly giving the child such treats as sweets. Please do not fall into the trap of saying that you know other people's children eat just as much as your child and yet are as skinny as rakes, and therefore that diet is not important. I will consider shortly some of the other reasons one child is obese when another isn't, but whatever the cause eating too much will aggravate it. Ignore other children. We are here only concerned with yours, and whatever the cause of his obesity he must be eating more than he needs.

Why does overeating occur? After all if people only ate to satisfy their hunger then there would be no problem. I have already discussed how some parents virtually train their children to overeat. The other potent cause is the way food is used as a pacifier. A study of over three thousand children in America revealed that almost 25 per cent of mothers used foods as rewards for good behaviour, 10 per cent used food deprivation as punishment, and 29 per cent used food as a pacifier. Favourite items were sweets, biscuits, and cake – perhaps the most fattening treats of all.

This use of food as a reward inevitably results in the child, and later the adult, using food in a similar way. If I feel I've done something well, or if I feel down and depressed, I often help myself to some special snack. I bet you do something similar. There is certainly a very high chance that you do something similar for your children. I know a number of doctors and nurses who keep a small supply of sweets to give to children who have behaved well when having an injection. Ignoring the arguments of the dentists against this for a moment, it is a classic example of food being given as a reward – not because nutrition is needed.

Constantly eating snacks between meals is a very important cause of obesity. Most really fat children are always eating. You can often spot them in the street, tube of sweets, or bag of crisps, in hand. Parents may mistakenly think that because their child is large he needs more food, whereas – of course – he is large because he has taken too much.

One final cause of overeating that can sometimes cause fatness is what the psychologists call 'sibling rivalry'. If a brother or sister is given a second helping of food, a child may feel that he must have the same, to keep level, whether he wants it or not!

The amount of energy a child uses up to balance the intake depends on how active he is, but activity is not the whole answer. The very lethargic, slow child is far less likely to burn up the Calories than a child who is constantly on the go. A particularly important group who tend to be inactive are the handicapped. Many parents make the mistake of giving these children extra food as some sort of compensation for their other difficulties, but this only worsens their situation.

One of the problems with working out how important activity is in obesity is trying to decide which is the chicken and which is the egg. In other words, does obesity cause inactivity, or does inactivity cause obesity? One thing that is known is that the body's metabolic rate – the speed with which the body uses up energy – is increased by exercise. Indeed the metabolic rate can even be affected by how much you eat, which shows just how confusing this whole subject is. In a classic series of experiments that were first performed in 1902 were repeated in 1922, and have recently been re-discovered, several individuals varied their daily food consumption by as much as 50 per cent. Despite this their weights remained relatively constant. It seems that their metabolism speeded up to compensate for the extra food. The opposite also seems to apply. The more you diet, the more your metabolism slows down. This could well explain why dieting so frequently fails, but all is not lost as increased exercise will increase the metabolic rate again. Exercise seems to be far more important in the shedding of weight than used to be realized.

You are probably thoroughly confused now, and if so, you are not alone. It is still reasonable to summarize current views on obesity by saying 'eat less and exercise more', but a great deal of research is constantly going on into the whole vexatious matter of why some people are obese and others aren't. Relevant factors probably include the family you are born into, the presence of brown fat, body type and even such strange factors as the season and the geography of where you live. Let us look at these one at a time.

The role of the family is extremely tricky to unravel. There is no doubt that fat parents have fat children; indeed, over 80 per cent of obese children have overweight parents, and if one child is fat the chances are that the second child will be fat too, though usually not as heavy as the first child. A study in America found that by the age of seventeen the children of two fat parents were three times as fat as the children of two lean parents.

All this seems to suggest a genetic cause, in the same way that parents who are fair-haired have fair-haired children. Indeed, a study in Denmark looked at whether adopted children took after their adoptive parents or their biological parents when it came to obesity. The answer was clear-cut. There was a very strong relationship between the body mass of children with their natural parents, and no relationship at all with their adoptive parents. This didn't just apply to obesity, but across the whole range of body fatness – from very thin to very fat. However, genetics are never the entire answer. For instance, overweight people are more likely to choose another overweight person as a marriage partner. The two parents will probably have similar attitudes to food, serving and eating more than slimmer parents. Their obvious enjoyment of food will not be missed by their children. Indeed patterns of eating, timing of meals, food preferences, speed of eating, and amount of exercise taken all reflect the attitudes of the parents and will be picked up by the children and then reinforced.

Studies on twins have shown that the child's environment is initially far more important than his genes, but over the age of ten the influence of heredity enlarges. However the research that showed wonderfully clearly how important the home environment is in obesity also revealed that not only do fat adults have fatter than average children – they also have fatter than average dogs!

Apart from the genes the family has an effect on obesity in other ways. Studies of large numbers of obese children show up parents on average older than the parents of non-obese children. Obesity also seems commoner among the children of divorced or separated parents. The highest incidence of childhood obesity is in one-parent families, and dwindles as family size increases. Perhaps the more children there are, the less food each manages to get at mealtimes!

In summary then it is clear that both lifestyle and genes are important when it comes to causing obesity. What we eat, as well as who we are, affects our risk of becoming obese. However, the one thing that we clearly do inherit from our parents is our basic shape. There are three well-recognized physical shapes. These are:

Ectomorph: Ectomorphs are long-limbed with narrow hands, fingers, and feet. These are the least likely to become overweight.

Mesomorph: This shape is the well-proportioned body, and mesomorphs do have to balance their energy expenditure with their food intake to maintain their correct weight.

Endomorph: Endomorphs have the greatest problem with weight control. They are short-limbed with broad feet and hands, and stubby fingers.

One of the most important recent discoveries in obesity research has been brown fat. This is a special type of fat that we are all born with, and the more we have of it the more efficiently we can burn off excess Calories – the Calories are literally turned to heat. Well before brown fat was discovered it had been shown that if healthy young people were deliberately overfed by 1300 Calories a day, their weight rose by 1 or 2 kilograms in the first ten days but not further. After that the extra food was dissipated as heat. It is possible that the child who gets fat is less able to turn Calories to heat, maybe because they have less brown fat. As yet, nothing can be done to increase the amount of brown fat a given individual possesses.

However unfair it may seem that some people have less than others, remember that obesity will not occur unless too much food is eaten.

There are several other factors that seem to affect childhood obesity, some of which seem easily explained. For instance the fact that obesity is commoner in the lower social classes is probably linked with poor diet. It is also reasonable to suggest that weight gain in winter and spring is connected with decreased opportunities for activity. Children in densely populated urban areas are more likely to be obese than children in rural areas, and white children are more likely to be obese than black children. Studies of immigrants to the USA show that the prevalence of obesity is increased in recent immigrants, and falls to levels comparable with the general population after three generations. Yet again this seems to be evidence that what you eat and how you live are far more important than your genetic inheritance.

I have already briefly mentioned the way that parents use food as a pacifier for their children. There is no doubt that children do the same for themselves. The unhappy child, especially around the age of seven or eight when he is beginning to break his tight emotional ties with his parents, often resorts to eating sweets or savoury snacks when he finds it difficult to make close friends with other children. Similarly some children who worry a lot, particularly about schoolwork, turn to food as a comfort. The child who becomes overweight then runs into new problems. Because he is overweight he will tend to exercise less. He may also be teased about his size, and this teasing may lead to further overeating. The old clichés about fat people being jolly and happy are often a very long way from the truth.

Ideally the way to deal with obesity is to prevent it. If you and your partner are overweight, then you will have realized that your child is at risk. The dietary guidelines given in Chapter 1 should have helped prevent your child becoming fat. In particular, increasing your child's fibre intake may well make him feel full sooner, without gaining too much weight. Plenty of exercise and a reduction in snacks will help considerably too.

If your child is already obviously overweight then what can you do about it? A slimming diet is unfortunately nowhere near as straightforward as it sounds. Is your child going to be expected to eat differently from the rest of the family? You may know yourself how hard it is for a well-motivated adult to stick to a diet. Think how much harder it is for a reluctant child.

The chief rule to remember if your child is overweight is that he must be eating more Calories than he needs, even if that is fewer than some of his slimmer friends. A regular intake of only one or two hundred Calories a day over his requirement may make him gain about a stone a year. This list of foods will show you just how little extra he may be eating, and therefore how little you may have to cut down.

1 glass (250 ml) of Coca Cola	100 Calories
1 glass (250 ml) of milk	160 Calories
1 Mars Bar	265 Calories
1 bag of crisps	160 Calories
1 portion of chips (6 oz)	600 Calories
1 chocolate digestive biscuit	135 Calories

Children often favour any of these as snacks and when you consider that as an alternative your child could eat an apple, which contains an average 50 Calories, or an orange, which has an average 40 Calories, and you can immediately see where some Calories savings can be made.

Perhaps most important when considering how your

child can best lose weight is that you are doomed to failure if he does not want to lose it. It is vital to get him to state that he really does want to lose weight, and is not just going along with your views. The other essential is to make sure that he does not feel he is being punished. If he is on a strict diet while the rest of the family tucks into cakes, chips, and chocolate, then he has every reason to feel annoyed and resentful. The whole family should have a similar diet, and the great thing about following the dietary advice in Chapter 1 is that it is excellent for the whole family, whether they are trying to lose weight or not. If your child is really very obese, you can try the trick of serving the same food as the rest of the family, but using a smaller plate.

When trying to reduce the total number of Calories your child eats, do remember that the word 'total' is important. If he occasionally goes to friends and eats Calorie-laden foods then it is not the end of the world. You simply need to reduce the Calorie count of the next few meals very slightly, and you will have compensated for his binge. To expect him to go to a birthday party and not join in is cruelty in the extreme.

The increasing number of low-Calorie, special dietetic foods on the market pose another dilemma. Is it sensible to feed your child with a diet of these? In general, it is inadvisable as this will keep him enthusiastic for, as an example, very sweet foods. It is far better for him to develop a taste for the healthier more natural foods, rather than a synthetic substitute. Having said that, I certainly prefer low Calories squashes to ordinary fruit squash drinks, although water is perhaps still the best drink of all. In the real world, children are going to ask for sweetened fruit drinks and the Calorie content of a glass of squash (80 Calories per half pint) is so high that saving these Calories is well worthwhile.

It is sensible to restrict eating to a single room in the house. The habit of eating snacks while watching television is asking for trouble. Children can easily sit glassy-eyed staring at the TV as they unthinkingly stuff crisps, biscuits, and the like into their mouths. If food is restricted to the kitchen or dining room, you may endure complaints but the advantages will be tremendous – not least to the previously crisp-covered carpet in the living room. Obviously it is unfair if the whole family does not follow this rule.

Exercise is important, although I certainly don't mean that you need to invest in a tracksuit and aerobics lessons for your child. Such simple exercise as a walk every day for twenty minutes or so will pay great dividends. Running around in the garden or riding a bike will do just as well. Anything is preferable to sitting still. There is considerable evidence that children now live a much more sedentary existence than they did in, for instance, the 1930s. This is largely the result of not having to walk to and from school, and also the time spent watching television. What is interesting is that the average daily intake of food for teenage boys in the 1930s was about 3100 Calories per day. It is now 2300 Calories per day. The fact that more boys are fat despite this reduction in intake of food goes some way to showing that importance of exercise in controlling weight.

One of the problems of helping children lose weight is that the child himself may see little advantage from the loss, even if you know the long-term advantages may be immense. This is where some kind of reward system – such as a star chart – may help. A star chart is simply a type of calendar on which you can stick coloured stars if your child achieves your targets for exercise or eating. It is of course vital that such targets are realistic. When your child gets stars on three days in a row you can offer him a small reward. You will find this works infinitely better than the threat of punishment for not keeping to the diet or taking exercise.

If your child fails to lose weight, despite his genuinely wanting to, then get him to keep a food diary, with your help. In this he should record every scrap of food that passes his lips, including snacks, biscuits, and sweets – and particularly all drinks. It usually becomes fairly obvious where the problem lies and where improvements can be made.

More dramatic aids, such as 'slimming tablets', are rarely helpful in childhood, and the ultimate intervention of hospital admission is of very limited value. Children who do not lose weight and who claim to be keeping to a diet almost always lose weight rapidly on hospital admission, because in hospital their diet and activity can be very closely supervised. However almost all regain their lost weight fairly rapidly on discharge from hospital. It certainly should be avoided if possible. However, your doctor or health visitor will offer advice if you are seriously worried about your child's weight problem, or else will be able to put you in touch with an interested paediatrician, so do ask for their help and advice.

In summary, here are a few basic guidelines to help your child lose weight.

- Remember that obesity is the result of more Calories being eaten than are used up by that particular child.
- You can only help your child if he wants to be helped. He must be an interested and willing partner in your plans.
- Try and plan high-fibre, low-Calorie meals for the whole family, offering the overweight child slightly smaller portions if necessary. On a smaller plate a small portion may look very generous.

- Avoid crisps, chocolate, sweets and biscuits between meals. If snacks are essential, then offer fruit.
- If your child wants a lot of snacks, try and find out why.
- Restrict eating to the kitchen or dining room – for the whole family.
- Encourage the whole family to exercise. Walks together are a good start.
- Try and slow down the speed at which your child eats, and allow plenty of time for chewing.
- Avoid sweet drinks, and try to encourage your child to drink water.
- Remember that most convenience foods are high in Calories, low in fibre, and frequently eaten much too quickly.
- If the problem is severe and responding poorly, then give as much encouragement as possible – possibly with a visual method such as a star chart.

Finally, remember how much easier prevention is than cure, and how many problems you will save your child later in his life if you watch his weight now.

9

Sickness and Diseases

'It's the same every Monday morning. Darren comes downstairs looking like death warmed up. He's always complaining of stomach ache, though the doctor can't find anything much wrong with him. If he's in pain, surely there must be something wrong. I know he doesn't enjoy school, and I sometimes wonder if that's the answer.'

So far this book has dealt mainly with the problems faced by the parents of healthy, albeit occasionally awkward, children. However, all children have episodes of illness. Tummy upsets, stomach aches, and constipation are all very common and can cause parents a great deal of concern, frequently quite needlessly. This chapter will look at all these problems, along with diarrhoea, vomiting, worms, and other related complaints.

The whole question of how to feed the child who is generally unwell needs to be considered first. When he is ill with flu, tonsilitis, or measles does it make any difference what you give him to eat or drink? Do you feed him or starve him? Does it matter?

Obviously any suggestions I give here must be general, and supplement any more specific advice your doctor may give you. However, there are some rules that are well worth observing.

Unless you are told anything to the contrary, your child does not need to eat anything that he doesn't want, and he can have anything that he wants. Please note the use of the word 'can', not 'must'. Parents stay in control. It is essential that you don't try and force your child to eat any particular foods. Instead you should use temptation and persuasion.

Most children's appetites are reduced by illness, and it is infinitely preferable to offer small quantities of favourite foods rather than trying to get them to eat normal-size meals. Occasionally you may find your child develops a slight stomach upset, with diarrhoea, when taking antibiotics. If this happens, it occurs because the antibiotic has also killed off some of the natural bacteria that live in the bowel. Giving live yogurt can sometimes help restore the normal balance of bacteria and control the symptoms.

It is also important that your child has plenty to drink when he is ill. Particularly with feverish illnesses, he will be sweating a great deal even if he is not passing much urine. The fluid lost in sweat needs to be replaced, and you should aim to give two to three pints a day for a pre-school child. It is no good offering large glasses or cups of fluid, unless this is what he asks for. Instead, you should offer small quantities of an assortment of drinks. It doesn't matter if he has water, milk, squash, fruit juices, or whatever. All fluid is useful, and it is sensible to offer what he will drink. The advice for children with diarrhoea is slightly different and I will return to that topic shortly. The child who is reluctant to drink may sometimes be tempted if he is allowed to drink through a straw.

Two common illnesses cause particular problems when it comes to eating and drinking, for very obvious reasons. These are sore throats and mumps. The child with a sore throat may well complain that swallowing is extremely painful, and you will find cold drinks or even ice lollies go down much easier. Sloppy foods, such as scrambled egg, macaroni cheese, yogurts, ice-creams, and soups all are far easier to swallow than toast, biscuits, and burgers. Warm drinks can also be tremendously soothing. All of my family loves hot blackcurrant juice as a treatment for colds and sore throats – perhaps because it is so expensive that we reserve it as a special treat!

Mumps makes swallowing unpleasant too. The glands chiefly affected are the parotid glands, which produce saliva. Eating or drinking normally leads to an increase in saliva production, as does even thinking about or smelling food. As a result any of these activities can worsen the pain of mumps. The pain may itself make the jaws feel stiff, and the stiffness can lead to worsening pain. It's a particularly miserable condition to have.

The best treatment is to offer a pain-killer, such as paracetamol elixir, and to give plenty of drinks. As soon as your child feels like eating, offer sloppy foods that will not need much chewing. Avoid offering sweets. Sucking sweets will lead to more production of saliva, and this will be even more painful. It is also vital, and comforting, to ensure that the mouth and teeth are kept clean. The teeth can become very coated with plaque and decay can readily set in without frequent brushing and rinsing.

After almost any illness, the first sign of recovery is the child becoming hungry again. The most sensible course from here is to return gradually to the normal healthy mixed diet that he usually eats. Some children take quite a long time to get their appetite back, while others are ravenously hungry almost at once! With this wide variation, I can offer no set guidelines for returning to a normal diet, but – in general if you trust your child to tell you how he feels and what he fancies, you won't go far wrong.

Diarrhoea and Vomiting

Any consideration of these extremely common problems in childhood must start with a brief summary of the normal anatomy and working of the bowel. Food initially enters the stomach, where acids and other digestive juices are mixed with the food, and the powerful muscular walls of the stomach help pulp it. The food then passes through a valve, the pyloric sphincter, into the small intestine. Here further enzymes in the digestive juices help to break down the food even further and the rhythmic contractions of the bowel help to propel it along. Here the majority of nutrients are absorbed into the bloodstream through the wall of the bowel. This is not smooth, but is covered with thousands of tiny *villi*, which are finger-like projections, and have the effect of greatly increasing the surface area of the bowel wall. The greater the surface area, the more nutrients can be absorbed.

In the large intestine fluid is absorbed from the motions, and the residue of indigestible matter is propelled towards the rectum where it is stored until an appropriate time, and opportunity, for it to be passed out through the anus.

That is what happens when everything is functioning normally, but with gastroenteritis the situation changes dramatically. Gastroenteritis simply means irritation and inflammation of the digestive tract. By far the commonest cause in affluent countries is infection by a virus, but there are other possible causes. Infection can also result from eating a food contaminated by bacteria, or by eating toxic substances such as might be found in toadstools, or even by eating foods to which you are allergic. Bacteria, hundreds of millions of them, are normally found in the bowel. Anything that changes the natural bacterial population of the bowel can also trigger an episode of gastroenteritis. This includes foreign travel, or at least eating foreign foods, and antibiotic drugs.

Whatever the cause, and it is usually irrelevant to the management, gastroenteritis is extremely common. The symptoms may be anything from mild nausea to profuse diarrhoea and vomiting. Sometimes stomach cramps, fever, and severe weakness may accompany the other symptoms, but in most people they fade away within forty-eight hours.

Gastroenteritis in adults and older children is a miserable inconvenience. In babies it can be fatal. The younger a child is with this condition the more serious it is. In England and Wales it accounts for approximately 10 per cent of all paediatric admissions to hospital, and in 1979 was reported as causing up to three hundred deaths annually. Under the age of two, dehydration can set in very rapidly, though with older children and adults the condition has to be severe and go on for a long time for this to occur.

The first line in treatment is to prevent the chief hazard, dehydration. If a child is dehydrated the eyes look glazed and sunken, and the mouth and tongue are dry. If in doubt call a doctor, and with diarrhoea and vomiting in under-twos you should *always* contact a doctor. In addition call a doctor if there is any blood in the motion. It helps if you can save some of the motion for the doctor to see, as it will help in reaching a diagnosis.

Obviously not all diarrhoea is caused by gastroenteritis. Other infection, such as ear or throat infections, can cause loose motions, as can worry. Whether it needs taking seriously or not depends on how your child is otherwise. If he is drinking normally and looks well, you can ignore it. If he is unwell or is vomiting, then you need medical help.

Most medication that has been used in the past to treat diarrhoea is either useless or potentlally dangerous. Many treatments are about as much help as that recommended a hundred years ago by the President of the New York Medical Society. He suggested plugging the rectum with beeswax and oil cloth! Obviously this might appear to stop the diarrhoea, but has absolutely no effect on the cause, or what is happening inside the abdomen.

Drugs such as Kaolin are almost as useless, and more powerful drugs such as Lomotil may even be dangerous. They work by slowing the bowel down and stop the diarrhoea leaving your system. However, they can have no effect on preventing the fluid accumulating in the intestine. Giving your child drugs like this may make you feel better – in that your child's diarrhoea may seem to stop – but is not doing any real good. Your child is still losing water and salts from his blood into the intestine, but you don't know about it and feel falsely reassured. They also stop the viruses or bacteria from being expelled from the bowel, and can have dangerous chemical effects – leading to severe muscular spasms.

So, what should you do with a child who has diarrhoea, but is not bad enough to need a doctor? Remembering that the hazard is dehydration, the answer is: give fluids. For a child who is drinking normally there is really no problem. Children who are reluctant to drink or eat or who have profuse diarrhoea should be given special mixtures which contain dextrose and just the right amount of chemicals. These are marketed as Dioralyte or Rehidrat, are available on prescription, or from chemist's shops, and consist of sachets of powder which should be mixed with the specified amounts of water. If you cannot obtain these, if you are on holiday for instance, Coca Cola diluted to half strength makes a very good substitute. As a guide you should aim to give 150 to 200 ml of fluid per kilogram of body weight per day. If kilograms still confuse you, a typical five-year-old boy weighs 18 kg (40 lb) and so should receive about three litres of fluid a day (approximately five pints). A child who is vomiting is best given the fluid in frequent small quantities.

A child with a fever requires even more fluid. For every two degrees Fahrenheit that his temperature goes up, his needs increase by 10 per cent. Such fluid replacement has become the mainstay of the treatment of gastroenteritis, and simple as it seems it is a lifesaver in the treatment of infants. Antibiotics are usually worse than useless.

As children recover, and begin to feel well enough to eat, it is best to start them on a fairly bland diet. It is also worth giving foods that do not need much chewing. Chewing can often start the nausea and retching off again.

In summary then . . .

- Most diarrhoea is caused by virus infections.
- If your child is otherwise well, you can ignore diarrhoea.
- You should ask for advice if he seems ill, has griping pains, has lost his appetite, or is vomiting.
- Most medication is at best useless and at worst dangerous.
- It is essential to offer adequate fluids.

Despite following all this advice, diarrhoea may occasionally persist for more than two or three days. Perhaps the most common cause for this is lactose intolerance. Lactose is the sugar in milk, and sometimes the virus will destroy the intestine's ability to digest and absorb it. If it is not absorbed it can itself cause diarrhoea. In other words, even though the original cause of the diarrhoea has gone, the symptom continues. If this is the case, stop milk, and all lactose-containing products such as cheese, butter, and so on. Your doctor or health visitor can give more complete guidance on lactose containing foods if necessary. Once the lactose is removed temporarily from the diet, both the diarrhoea and intestine recover, though it may take several weeks of milk avoidance before the condition clears completely.

If diarrhoea goes on for more than four or five days, then your doctor might also ask you to collect a small sample of the motion for analysis in the laboratory. Occasionally diarrhoea is caused by bacteria that are helped by antibiotics. A bacteria known as campylobacter, which may be caught from pets, can cause diarrhoea and is easily cured by the antibiotic Erythromycin. However, as antibiotics may make more forms of diarrhoea worse, rather than better, doctors will want to know exactly which bacteria they are dealing with, rather than guessing. Hence the need for a specimen.

There are other occasional causes for loose motions. I have already mentioned anxiety and tension, but excessive drinking of fruit juices, or sugary liquids might produce diarrhoea as may weaning foods such as apple puree or mashed banana which have high levels of fructose and are worth bearing in mind. Indeed, there is a small but definite group of children, usually between the age of six months and two years, who have persistent diarrhoea but are otherwise perfectly well. Paediatricians often call this toddler diarrhoea 'the peas and carrots syndrome' for obvious reasons. Provided they are fit and otherwise healthy, and are growing normally, such children are not a cause for concern. Your doctor may ask to test the motions to exclude certain infections or conditions like coeliac disease, but if these are normal it usually recovers spontaneously.

Vomiting

Vomiting is frequently an accompaniment to diarrhoea, and the management is as discussed earlier. However, it may occur alone, or as part of another illness. Almost anything may start it, from a simple cold, to tonsilitis, ear infections, and so on. Simple vomiting does not usually last more than six to eight hours. If a baby is sick for longer than this, ask your doctor's advice, sooner if he has diarrhoea, or if an older child doesn't keep drinks down for twelve hours you should seek help.

When treating a child who is vomiting, remember that small sips of fluid are easier to keep down than big drinks. Coca Cola, or similar drinks, also seem to stay down more easily, but are best given flat rather than fizzy. These drinks are available almost everywhere in the world, so can solve your treatment problem if you are away on holiday.

One other common reason for vomiting is travel sickness. With luck you should be able to avoid this by ensuring your child can see out of the window, using a booster seat if necessary, does not spend the journey looking down at toys or books, and by avoiding large meals or drinks just before the journey. Small dry snacks, such as biscuits, are helpful, as are sweets that can be sucked. Distractions in the form of stories or songs on cassette tapes can help a great deal, but if all else fails have a word with your doctor or pharmacist about suitable travel sickness pills.

Worms

For some reason, the realization that a child has worms often makes parents ashamed, guilty, and worried. There is absolutely no need. Almost every family gets them at some time, and they are not a sign of a dirty or unhygienic household. Any child can get worms, and if yours does, then consider it as a trivial nuisance that can easily be cured.

The commonest type is threadworms. These appropriately look like little lengths of white thread, and can sometimes be seen in the motions or around the anus. If a doctor suspects the diagnosis he may suggest that you stick a piece of sellotape over the anus at bedtime. If the worms appear overnight they will stick to the tape and be clearly visible in the morning. Incidentally, don't make the mistake that one parent I know of made. She gave her child bananas for the first time, and then noticed the little black threads that are part of the banana when they appeared in a nappy and assumed they were worms!

The only symptom that threadworms can cause is itching around the anus, when the female comes out of the anus to lay her eggs. Sometimes vaginal itching may occur, if the worms have been transferred by scratching, and bedwetting may also result from the irritation. However, the itching is the only real symptom. Threadworms do not cause tiredness, tummy ache, weight loss, or any of the hundred and one other symptoms that have been attributed to them. When the child scratches he transfers some eggs to his fingernails, and these may then be passed on to others, or he may reinfest himself by putting his hands to his mouth.

Treatment is simple. Your doctor or pharmacist can provide special tablets or medicine, such as Pripsen (Piperazine), or Vermox (Mebendazole). A single dose is usually enough, though it is wise to repeat this after two weeks. However it is absolutely essential that the whole family takes the treatment, or it may continue to be passed on. Reinfestation can also be prevented by keeping your child's nails cut short, and by getting him to wear pants at bedtime for a few nights to prevent scratching.

The other sorts of worms are much rarer. Roundworms are only common in tropical countries, and look like white earthworms. They live in the small intestine, often grow up to six inches long, and may occasionally be vomited out, although usually they are passed in the motions. They can also be cured by a single dose of the appropriate drug.

Tapeworms can occur in any country and are the result of eating undercooked pork. They are seen as flat, white segments that move about in the stool, and this is frequently the first sign of the infection although occasionally abdominal pain may be a problem. It goes without saying that you should make sure pork is always cooked fully.

Finally, in this rather unpleasant section, comes toxocara, a type of roundworm which infests cats and dogs. Children can become infected by playing with their own pets, or accidentally becoming contaminated by dog faeces when playing in a local park. It is quite absurd that dogs are allowed to defaecate in areas where children play.

Toxocara eggs are transferred from the child's hands to his mouth and then to the intestine where they hatch. The larvae penetrate through the bowel wall and can then be spread to any part of the body. Here the irritation they cause can result in diseases, even fits and blindness. Treatment can obviously kill the actual worms, but any disease that has already resulted may persist. Prevention is all-important. If you have a pet make sure that it is regularly dewormed.

Constipation

Everyone knows what constipation is. It is the infrequent passing of stools that are too hard. The problem lies in the definition of the words 'infrequent' and 'too hard'. All too many parents become unnecessarily worried about their children's bowel habits, all because somewhere along the line they have got the idea that motions must be passed regularly every day.

Think back to my description of the anatomy of the bowel and how it functions. The motions collect in the rectum. When the rectum is full, the brain becomes aware of this, and provided the child has an opportunity to go to the toilet there are no problems.

However, problems can, and do, arise if this natural pattern is interfered with. There are three main causes of this – pain, lack of opportunity to pass a motion, and the use of laxatives.

The first two are straightforward. The third may surprise you. If passing a motion is painful, the child will obviously be reluctant to do so. The commonest reason for pain is an anal fissure, a tiny crack in the lining of the anus which understandably causes discomfort when a motion passes it. Usually started by a very hard motion, a vicious circle of pain causing constipation causing pain can easily be set up. This is one of the few occasions when a gentle laxative may help. Some doctors may also offer a local anaesthetic ointment to use before and after passing a motion.

The lack of an appropriate opportunity to pass a motion may also cause problems. The commonest reason for this is embarrassment at school. A child may be worried about asking permission to go to the toilet and so does not go when he should: the body then gradually learns to ignore the messages from the rectum that it is full. I even recall one child who was reluctant to go to the toilet at school as he was so frightened of the 'crunchy loo paper'.

However, by far the greatest cause of constipation is the use of laxatives. If a parent mistakenly believes a child to be constipated and gives laxatives, the bowel will empty before it is full. The normal reflexes will be lost. If, for example, a mother gives a dose of laxative on a Friday because the child has not passed any motions since Tuesday he will certainly pass a substantial movement, so confirming to the parent that the laxative was needed. However the rectum will now be abnormally empty and the child will not go for several days again. Before he has a chance to go, a second dose of laxative may be given. The cycle is set up, and laxatives may be used for the next seventy years!

All this can be avoided if you remember a few simple rules. Never give laxatives unless on a doctor's instructions. Remember that the bowel will empty itself naturally when it is ready, and the frequency of this varies tremendously. Sometimes a child may go three times in a day. On other occasions it may only be once every four days. It really doesn't matter. There is no need to worry about toxins being absorbed into the system, or the child getting sluggish, or developing pains. Don't pester your child with questions as to how often he has gone and what the motion was like. The less it bothers you, the less it will bother him. There is absolutely no need for a child to go every day.

Any illness may make a child go less frequently. Again this does not matter. It is simply a result of his eating and exercising less, and may also ensue through fever leading to excess sweating. The motions for a couple of days afterwards may be firmer and larger, but this is of no consequence. If you really feel you have to do something, then extra fibre is all that is required.

I cannot stress enough that constipation is not an illness. If the child has other symptoms – such as bad breath – look for another cause. Doctors see far more problems caused by overconcern and abuse of laxatives than are ever caused by constipation.

One paradoxical result of chronic constipation is soiling. This occurs when a child regularly passes a motion in his pants or elsewhere, but not in the lavatory. Indeed he may even appear to have diarrhoea. What happens is that a plug of very hard faeces forms in the rectum and the only motions that can get past are soft, watery ones. The child may be reluctant to go to the toilet when he needs to, or it is a natural development of the toddler negativism that I discussed in Chapter 5. If your child begins to soil after he has achieved normal bowel control, do go and consult your doctor.

Pica

Pica is 'dirt eating'. It is relatively common between the ages of two and four when it only needs to be considered a problem if the child persistently eats dirt, coal, faeces, and other similar substances. Obviously all babies do this, but once they have discovered that something tastes revolting they don't try it again. My daughter went through a couple of days of putting snails in her mouth and chewing them when she was eighteen months old. She soon gave up!

Some doctors believe that children who are anaemic are more likely to eat dirt, and so may wish to take a blood test. However, pica is certainly not caused by worms and it is not a sign of mental or emotional problems (although it is commoner in the mentally handicapped).

If anaemia is ruled out or treated, the condition usually settles sooner or later. The only action you need take is to make sure that he does not have the opportunity to eat things that are poisonous. If he chews wood, at least make sure it is not covered with lead paint.

Professor Ronald Illingworth of Sheffield University once listed the following 'foods' that he has known children eat: dirt, rags, splinters, wallpaper, ashes, paper, plaster, match heads, shoestrings, sand, hair, rubber, coal, stones, toys, buttons, clothes, soap, thread, sticks, worms, bugs, faeces, polish, oilcloth, filth from the dust-bin, crayons, wood, celluloid – and so on, and on. It is an amazing list, and worrying too when you realize that some of the substances are poisonous. Indeed, nearly seven out of ten children admitted to hospital with poisoning are also dirt eaters. If your child shows an inclination to eat unsuitable things, do discuss it with your doctor.

Tummy Ache

Abdominal pains are an extremely common feature of childhood. However, not all 'tummy aches' are abdominal pains. A short while ago I saw a child of three who was complaining of tummy ache. When I asked her to show me where it hurt, she pointed to her ear. 'Tummy ache' for her simply meant 'pain'. For other young children it means only that they don't feel well. Do make sure you know what your child means, as adults and children don't always speak the same language.

Sudden severe abdominal pain needs assessment by a doctor. It may be caused by a huge number of conditions, and frequently is caused by infection elsewhere in the body. For instance, children with tonsilitis often develop swollen glands in the abdomen that cause pain, and there is no need to be surprised if your doctor diagnoses a cause that doesn't seem to have anything to do with the abdomen.

However, the tummy ache that keeps recurring is another problem altogether. The National Child Development Study examined eleven thousand seven-year-olds and found that 15 per cent had recurrent abdominal pains, and another study of school children in Bristol showed 11 per cent were sufferers. One of the commonest symptoms of childhood to get referred to hospital specialists, it causes so many problems to doctors, not to mention parents and children, that an entire medical book is devoted to the subject.

If your child does have recurrent stomach pains that cause you or him concern, then do consult your doctor. There are many possible causes – an article in the *British Medical Journal* listed a minimum of forty-two – but it is generally accepted that in around 95 per cent no physical cause will be found. Even though this obviously makes it less likely that your doctor, or a hospital paediatrician, will be able to name a specific cause, it is nonetheless essential that a cause is searched for. The doctor may want to arrange a few investigations, and almost certainly will want to examine a urine specimen to exclude an infection. It saves time to take a specimen along with you.

If a specific cause is found, then treatment can follow. However, what do you do if your child is one of the 95 per cent in whom no cause is found?

Such children are typically of primary school age, at which point boys are affected to the same degree as girls. For older children, particularly nearing puberty, more girls are affected. Many of the children are clearly very tense and anxious, and it is generally thought that the vast majority of pains are psychosomatic. In other words they are caused by emotional stress.

It is essential to be aware of two points about psychosomatic abdominal pains. First of all, parents and doctors should never diagnose this as the cause simply because they cannot find another, physical, cause. There must be some positive evidence of stress – whether in the home, school, or elsewhere. Often this will be glaringly apparent, as in the child who only gets tummy ache on one particular day of the week, and only in term time. On other occasions the stresses will be less obvious, but are nonetheless worth searching for.

The other fact you must remember is that psychosomatic pains are *not* imaginary. They are as real as the pains of appendicitis. Doubtless you occasionally get headaches, particularly after a stressful day. The pain of the headache is often severe, but I am sure you would accept that – however closely a doctor examined your head – there is no major physical cause for it. It is the same with the recurrent abdominal pains of childhood that are caused by tension.

The analogy with headaches is particularly appropriate. Children with recurrent tummy ache often have a family history of headaches, migraine, and so on. I have little doubt that some of these are psychosomatic symptoms, but there is a definite group for whom the trigger of the pain – whether in the head or stomach – is a food allergy. I will look at the whole topic of food allergies in Chapter 11, but meanwhile it is well worth keeping your eyes open to note whether your child gets his symptoms after any particular food. Milk is a frequent culprit, but there is a danger of becoming obsessed with looking for an allergic cause, rather than facing up to a psychological cause that is all too obvious to someone else.

It helps to be able to explain to a child why he feels pain when he is tense. You will recall from the start of this chapter that food is moved along the bowel by waves of muscular contraction. These waves cannot normally be felt, but tension makes the waves more powerful and also intensifies any physical symptom. When you are frightened and anxious, for instance, your heart beats faster. Most people then become aware of this thumping, even though they normally don't notice their heart beat. This increased awareness of feelings, plus the increasing muscular spasms of the bowel, can all lead to the sensation of pain. If you, or your doctor, can get this idea over to your child in a simple manner, he will be much less concerned.

If this alone is not enough, other treatments of recurrent abdominal pain of course depend on the cause. Many parents are greatly reassured to know that there is no serious physical cause such as the mythical condition of 'grumbling appendicitis'. The reassurance lowers the emotional temperature in the family, and often the pains gradually fade away. Parents should, of course, consult the doctor again if the nature of the pain changes.

Mild painkillers can help if the pain seems to be distressing the child. Laxatives are generally useless. In the long run, many children with abdominal pains continue to get these, or headaches, as adults. The condition never kills, or does any serious harm. The less fuss that you make about the symptoms the better. Be sympathetic, accept that it is real, exclude possible food triggers, look for stresses, and remember that it is otherwise harmless once a doctor has checked your child over.

Allergies and Additives

'Sometimes when I read the labels on some of the packets of food that I buy, I am worried sick by the list of chemicals and additives. Are they harmful? What effects will they have on our children?'

Few topics to do with childhood nutrition cause as much controversy as allergies and additives. On the one hand certain self-help groups claim that a majority of childhood behaviour problems result from chemical additives, while on the other some of the more conservative paediatricians dismiss the topic almost completely.

One of the great difficulties in any discussion of food allergy is that different people often use the same words to mean different things. Take the word 'allergy' for instance. Many reactions that children might have to food are not true allergies at all. It is essential to understand what the various terms mean if you are to make any sense of articles you read, or of talks and broadcasts that you might hear.

So – what is an allergy? Whenever a potentially harmful chemical comes into contact with the body, the body's defences immediately produce protective chemicals. This happens with all of us. However in an allergic person the body mistakes a usually harmless substance for a harmful one and the protective reaction occurs inappropriately.

Any substance that triggers off this reaction is called an allergen, and the range of possible allergens is vast – ranging from pollens, through mites that are found in house dust, to drugs or foods.

The majority of children with allergies inherit this tendency. If both parents have allergies, there is a two out of three chance that their children will have allergies. If one parent has allergies and the other does not, then the children have a 25 to 50 per cent chance of being allergic, and if neither parent has allergies the risk for a child is around 10 per cent. Incidentally the children of allergic parents do not necessarily have the same type of allergy as their parents.

However, even if a child is allergic he or she won't have any symptoms until he has been exposed at least twice to the substances he's allergic to. On the first exposure the body may develop antibodies to the substance. These are very similar to the antibodies produced when the body is invaded by a virus or bacteria. In the case of allergies the particular antibody is an immunoglobulin called IgE. These antibodies are found in the lining of the nose, throat, lungs, skin and gut. When the allergen and the antibodies come into contact with each other, another chemical – histamine – is released. This dilates the blood vessels and makes their walls more porous. As a result normal tissue fluid leaks through and if the allergy is in, for example, the nose, the lining of the nose swells up, the nose runs, and so on. In the lungs an attack of asthma may be triggered, in the skin urticaria (or hives) may result, and in the bowel symptoms such as nausea, vomiting, abdominal pain and diarrhoea may occur, and sometimes nasal or chest symptoms may be triggered off. Whichever part of the body produces the symptoms is called the target organ.

I do not intend here to discuss all of the common

allergies. Indeed many excellent books have been devoted to allergies alone. While allergies may occur to items that are inhaled or touched, this chapter will only deal with allergens that a child might eat or drink. Why particular allergies occur is something of a mystery, but there is some evidence that exposing babies to particular foodstuffs too early in life may be part of the problem.

Throughout our lives, the walls of our intestines allow certain nutrients to pass through, keeping others in the bowel. In early infancy the bowel is less selective. Large proteins can pass through the bowel wall in the first three or four months, proteins that are up to ten times as large as those that can just about pass through at four to six months. These proteins may lead to antibody formation, and to full allergic reactions when the child is later exposed to these foodstuffs again. If the introduction of the food had been delayed till after six months of age, its proteins would not have passed through the bowel wall, the antibodies would not have been formed, and the allergy might not have occurred. Though still only a theory, this is plausible enough to constitute yet another argument to delay weaning, and mothers who have allergies would be wise to breast-feed for as long as possible – avoiding cow's milk 'top-ups' if they can.

So, how do you tell if your child has a food allergy? Listed in Table 3 are some of the conditions that have been associated with these allergies to foods. Please do remember that all these symptoms have many other possible causes, and allergy is only one. However, there are certain hints that will help you Spot if allergy is a likely problem. For a start it is essential to realize that if a particular symptom is caused by a food allergy it will occur on every occasion your child eats that food. If it only occurs sometimes, it is not an allergy.

If your family suffers from allergies (we call this an

Table 3 Childhood Conditions
that may be linked to Food Allergies

Eczema	Hayfever
Asthma	Migraine
Abdominal Pains	Diarrhoea
Acute swellings of mouth or tongue	Urticaria
Vomiting	Bloated Stomach
Conjunctivitis	

Recurrent coughs, runny noses, and ear infections and
the most serious, but mercifully rare, acute anaphylactic
shock.

atopic family) you will be particularly on the lookout for
allergic problems. Sometimes the answers will be obvious.
If your child comes out in a dramatic rash every time he
eats eggs, then an allergy is clear cut. What is less easy to
sort out is the possibility of allergy related to other
conditions. Some children, for instance, keep getting ear
infections. Sometimes this can be the result of an allergy
to cow's milk, but often it is not. How on earth do you
sort it out?

For a start it is well worth discussing the problem with
your family doctor, or – if necessary – a paediatrician. If
your suspicions of allergy are strong, take along a diary of
symptoms and food intake. The doctor may be able to
spot a link between foods that were taken before a specific
symptom occurred. Alternatively he may be able to diagnose some other, non-allergic, cause for your child's
symptoms.

Table 4 lists some of the foods that have been most
commonly implicated in allergic problems. A good dietary
history is perhaps the most important diagnostic test.
Blood tests can sometimes help the diagnosis, but are
most conclusive when there is already very strong evi-

Table 4 Main foods that have been
Implicated in Childhood Food Allergies

Milk	Egg
Wheat	Cheese
Fish	Chocolate
Tomato	Soya
Citrus Fruits	Yeast
Coffee	

dence from the dietary history. Skin tests, in which an allergen is injected into the skin and the reaction is observed, are rarely particularly specific although they can have a place. Unfortunately a positive reaction to a skin test does not necessarily prove the existence of a food allergy.

Perhaps the simplest way to confirm an allergy is to withdraw that particular food from your child's diet. It sounds simple enough anyway, and so it is if your child is only allergic to shrimps, or Coca Cola. But what if you suspect a milk allergy? To exclude milk completely means carefully examining the recipes or labels for many types of bread, cake, and convenience foods. This sort of diet needs detailed advice from an expert, and your doctor should be able to put you in touch with a qualified and interested dietician. Sometimes a major exclusion, or elimination, diet must be used. In this, your child's diet will be dramatically restricted over a period of time to see if there is any change to the symptom pattern.

It has been shown that the type of meat least likely to cause significant reactions is lamb, the least troublesome cereal is rice, and also that peeled potatoes, lettuce, and peeled pears are also very unlikely to start any form of reaction. Some dieticians advise initial exclusion diets based primarily around just these foods, with a gradual re-introduction of other foods when all symptoms have cleared. If such a strict diet is used, a multivitamin preparation is strongly advised. You can see that such a diet is extremely strict, time consuming, and awkward. You really do need to think carefully as to whether such a step is really worth it.

If excluding a suspected food leads to an apparent improvement in symptoms, that alone is not enough for the diagnosis of food allergy. It could just be coincidence. You really need to give the food again and see if symptoms return, and then withdraw it to see if he improves. If you don't apply this test you may deprive your child for years of a foodstuff that does him no harm at all.

Once you have finally decided that your child has a symptom that is the result of a food allergy, then what do you do about it? Avoidance of the food is ideal, but may be difficult or simply not worthwhile. An older child may decide that a fit of sneezing is a price he is prepared to pay for a slice of chocolate cake. You should not make the treatment worse than the problem.

If you decide that a strict diet is the answer for your child, then do ensure that his nutrition is otherwise satisfactory. One study looked at a group of twenty-three children with severe eczema who had failed to respond to conventional medications but had remained reasonably well on a milk-free diet. Unfortunately diet records showed that thirteen of the eczema group had significantly low calcium intakes – less than 75 per cent of the recommended daily amount. One of the children even eventually developed rickets. Strict diets can help but they can be hazardous, and you should get professional advice.

Drugs such as antihistamines may be useful if the reaction is a simple one such as an attack of hives after eating particular foods, but may be sedative and certainly aren't as good as avoiding the allergen in the first place. Another drug, disodium cromoglycate, which prevents histamine release, is promising but needs to be taken before eating the suspected food, which is not always easy.

If your child suffers from conditions such as eczema or migraine it is well worth getting more information on possible dietary triggers from your doctor or health visitor. If they cannot help, the self-help groups and other organizations listed in the appendix will almost always be able to offer advice. There is no guarantee that you will unearth a dietary cause, but it is well worth exploring the possibility.

You may by now have noticed that I have not mentioned some of the other so-called food allergies that you have heard of elsewhere. What about gluten sensitivity, or allergy to food additives?

The reason is quite simple. Though important, they are not true allergies. If you remember that an allergic reaction is a specific type of repeatable chemical reaction that always involves antibodies and allergens, all these other problems are better described as types of food intolerance. The word allergy should be reserved for true chemical allergies. Indeed this is more than just splitting hairs over definitions, as different problems require different approaches.

One of the commoner forms of food intolerance is lactose intolerance. Lactose is the natural sugar found in milk, and as I discussed in Chapter 9, temporary intolerance, or inability to digest it, not uncommonly follows episodes of diarrhoea in young children. The body is unable to deal with this particular sugar, but in no way is this an allergy. While lactose intolerance is usually temporary, gluten intolerance – or coeliac disease – is far more likely to be permanent. For sufferers from this condition the presence of gluten – part of wheat, rye, barley and oats – in the bowel leads to damage to the lining of the bowel which prevents other nutrients being absorbed. I will discuss coeliac disease in far more detail in the next chapter.

Another group of substances of which many children are intolerant are food additives. What was your immediate reaction to the phrase 'food additives'? Most people today think of additives as being entirely a bad thing, without which we would all be a lot better off. They have certainly become one of modern society's 'bad guys', being blamed for everything from behaviour disturbance in children to cancer. Indeed, if you were to read on a package that it contained additive E 300 you would possibly prefer to choose something more 'natural'.

Well, E 300 is vitamin C. By far the commonest food additives are sugar and salt, and there is no need to reach the automatic assumption that other chemical additives are a bad thing. They should all be treated in the same way as sugar and salt, in other words eaten in moderation realizing what excessive consumption can do to you.

Why are additives used at all? The simplest and most important reason is the dramatic change in the structure of society over recent decades. At the turn of the century over half the population of most Western countries was involved in food production. Today in the USA and UK the figure is nearer 5 per cent, as a result of which food must be transported further and processed or preserved to keep fresh longer. In the past the lack of preservatives meant extravagant waste, the need to purchase food daily, and the risk of eating infected and stale food. It is easy to forget in our passion for 'natural' products that you cannot get more natural than salmonella. Many health problems have actually been avoided by food additives.

In addition to preservatives, other additives such as emulsifiers, stabilizers, and thickeners are used to improve appearance and texture. Perhaps the least desirable additives are food colouring, since their only importance is in improving the appearance of foods, yet whenever companies experimentally introduce food without colouring agents, sales fall. One hopes that this pattern of purchasing will change with greater public awareness as colouring matter is really totally unnecessary and has been implicated in various problems – of which more later. Certainly when we used to holiday in France my children, after initial complaints, accepted happily that much French orange squash is a pale, dull (and colouring agent-free), but delicious drink. Given time one can only hope that other countries follow the French example.

Incidentally, not only packaged and preserved foods contain additives. Some fresh foods such as fruit are treated with chemicals which make them look more shiny and attractive and the skins of citrus fruits occasionally have colouring added. Even meat may contain chemicals or drugs that have originally been fed to the animals to encourage growth or suppress infections. Consumers need to know which foods contain these chemicals, and though voluntary provision of such information is now being offered by some of the more enlightened supermarket chains, legislation will be needed before we all know everything we ought to know about what we eat.

No one can hope to avoid all known chemical food additives unless they are totally self-sufficient in food production, not a realistic prospect for most of us. Try to consider when you shop why they are in the food you are purchasing. Are they there to improve the taste and condition of the food, or is their presence more to do with the manufacturer's convenience and marketing policy? Labelling laws have changed to make it easier for consumers to identify food additives. In the EC all foods either have to carry an E number or actual additive name in the ingredients list. The E numbers are not a secretive way of hiding information, but a logical way of presenting it. After all, it is infinitely easier to read or remember E 215 than 'Sodium ethyl para-hydroxybenzoate', provided one has a code to such numbers. Many supermarkets are now enlightened enough to provide booklets which give details of their labelling, E number codes, and so on, so that the modern consumer has more information than ever before on what he or she is actually buying and eating. In addition, in the references to this chapter I list publications which give the code to E numbers.

Ironically it can be extremely difficult to find out what colouring agents are in medications purchased over the counter, or on a doctor's prescription. I have on occasions had to find out if particular drugs contain certain colouring agents when treating sensitive patients. The pharmaceutical companies do provide the information on request, but the letters are frequently marked 'confidential'. I wonder why?

Having determined what food additives are, and what their purposes are, the question then arises as to whether they do any harm. There is no unequivocal answer, but I have little doubt that in some children certain additives do cause behavioural problems. I am equally certain that the majority of behaviour problems are not linked with food intolerance. It is much easier to blame multi-national food companies than it is to explore problems closer to home, but nevertheless I have come across very many cases where changes in the diet have helped.

Of all the behaviour problems that have been most implicated in the additive debate, hyperactivity is the most important. Hyperactive is a term that covers the child who is physically and mentally restless with boundless energy. Such children don't sit still, they talk a lot, and sleep very badly. They certainly exhaust their parents.

However, the diagnosis of hyperactivity is far from definite. For example the condition is supposed to be far more common in the United States than in Britain, a difference that probably reflects doctors' attitudes rather than children's health. Some doctors even dispute that the condition exists at all, although – to quote one mother who wrote to me – 'If you doubt they exist, just try having mine for a week.'

Numerous causes have been examined from what American doctors call 'minimal brain dysfunction', possibly dated from birth trauma, through lead poisoning – from petrol fumes and diet. In 1973, in California, one Dr Ben Feingold proposed that salicylates, artificial flavouring and food colouring were causes of hyperactivity. He produced two highly successful books advising diets and ways of avoiding these substances, and there did appear to be much anecdotal evidence to support his belief that a diet free of these substances helped. Since then the battle has raged, with papers regularly being published in the medical journals making claims and counter-claims. For example, one major article from the Institute of Psychiatry in London examined three reviews of the Feingold diet and concluded that any help obtained was largely a placebo response, while another report in the journal *Science* found definite impairment in the performance of learning tests when a group of hyperactive children received food colourings, although not when other 'normal' children received the colourings. The children had no idea whether they were receiving the colouring agents or not.

One of the most interesting British studies into this topic was published in 1993 and looked at a group of seventy-eight children, referred to a clinic because of hyperactive behaviour. These children were put on to a 'few foods' elimination diet, and a remarkable fifty-nine improved in behaviour during the trial. Even more remarkably, for nineteen of the children it was possible to perform a double blind trial. In other words neither the children nor their carers knew which foods were being taken. The problem foods caused impaired behaviour, and impaired psychological test performance. The authors of this academic paper concluded 'clinicians should give weight to the accounts of parents and consider this treatment in selected children with a suggestive medical history'. In particular they noted that the problem of irritability seemed to be very considerably improved.

By no means all hyperactive children will respond to diet, and there is little doubt that the debate is likely to continue for some time yet, but I think all the evidence suggests that a small but significant group of children with behaviour problems are affected adversely by food additives. As a result it is well worth trying such a diet, but the process is not easy, requires constant supervision, and carries the considerable danger that if it fails, certain parents may feel it is just because they are not trying hard enough and may put their child on stricter and stricter diets. Do not fall into this trap. If dietary change does not solve your child's behavioural or hyperactivity problem, then look for other causes and ways of helping. Do not let it become an obsession.

Detailed advice on the Feingold diet can be obtained from organizations that have been set up for hyperactive children. You will find an address in the appendix. However, not all children require a strict diet. Simply avoiding certain additives may be enough. I have evidence of a large number of children whose sleepless nights improved after a reduction in the amount of tartrazine (E 102) in their diet. This yellow colouring is found in a wide range of foods, such as orange, lime, and lemon squash, fizzy drinks, many packet convenience foods, salad cream, brown sauce, the coating of fish fingers, and so on. On the numerous occasions that I have discussed this chemical on TV or radio broadcasts, I have been inundated with messages from parents who have found that avoiding it helped their children.

The food additives that the Hyperactive Children's Support Group in the UK recommend should be avoided are listed in Table 5. When trying such exclusion diets

Table 5 Food Additives that the
Hyperactive Children's Support Group Advise Should be Avoided

E102	Tartrazine
E104	Quinoline Yellow
107	Yellow 2G
E110	Sunset Yellow FCF
E120	Cochineal
E122	Carmoisine
E123	Amaranth
E150	Caramel
E151	Black PN
154	Brown FK
155	Brown HT
E210	Benzoic Acid
E124	Ponceau 4R
E127	Erythrosine
128	Red 2G
E132	Indigo Carmine
E133	Brilliant Blue FCF
E211	Sodium benzoate
E220	Sulphur dioxide
E250	Sodium nitrate
E251	Potassium nitrite
E320	Butylated hydroxyamisole
E321	Butylated hydroxytoluene

persevere for at least three weeks, and don't overlook colouring agents in toothpaste and medicines. If it does seem to help, you can reintroduce additives one at a time until you identify the culprit or culprits. That is the one, or ones, to avoid.

No one can guarantee that an exclusion diet will help your child. Indeed it is impossible at present to tell if 1 per cent, 5 per cent, 25 per cent, or 100 per cent of children with behaviour problems or hyperactivity will benefit from such a diet. But it doesn't really matter; food colourings are completely unnecessary from any nutritional point of view, and if they cause problems for only one child in a thousand, then that is one too many.

Special Problems
and Special Diets

*'When the doctor told us our son was diabetic it felt
like the bottom had dropped out of our world. We
couldn't even begin to see how he would cope with
the special foods – not to mention the injections and
all that. We were horrified.'*

Father of 6-year-old

Whether by circumstance or by choice, some children
need special diets. The child of the vegetarian couple, the
diabetic teenager, and the child with coeliac disease all
need individual consideration. A book such as this
obviously cannot deal with every possible condition in
detail. However there are certain factors that are common
to many of the different conditions, and it is the general
principles that I will be covering here. If your child does
have an illness that requires a special diet, I would
strongly urge you to contact the organization that special-
izes in the problem. Such groups are listed in the appendix, and the help they can offer is invaluable.

As the parent quoted at the start of this chapter said, it
can seem to be a total disaster when you are told that your
child has a condition such as diabetes. After all, parents
have enough problems when their children are supposed

to be eating 'normally'. Almost every child uses tactics such as food refusal to get attention, assert independence, or just be a total nuisance. When the child has to be on a special diet, the potential for problems and for rebellion is that much greater.

With the child who has to eat a fairly strict diet, because of diabetes for instance, food refusal cannot be ignored in the same way it can for a healthy child. Such children often have to eat particular foods at particular times. As a result parents are likely to try all manner of ploys to persuade their child to eat, and failure may lead to tremendous feelings of guilt, anger, and resentment, not to mention despair. If the other parent, assuming there is one around, does not offer encouragement and assistance the obstacles may seem insurmountable. If you find you are getting into this sort of situation, do please seek professional advice from a dietician, health visitor, or doctor. The self-help groups have all got tremendous experience in helping other parents with similar problems, and can be a real source of strength.

Diabetes

The problems of diabetes result from a lack of insulin. Whenever food is eaten, insulin is released by the pancreas – a gland in the abdomen – to deal with the sugar in the food. Some of the sugar is immediately converted to energy, and the rest is stored in the liver as glycogen. The glycogen can be turned back into sugar when more energy is required.

If there is not enough insulin, sugar builds up in the blood as this conversion to glycogen does not take place. When the blood sugar level rises, sugar will eventually leak out into the urine. The chief symptoms tend to be increased thirst, increased output of urine, and generally feeling unwell. It can even lead to coma.

Diabetes is far more common in the elderly than in children. About 3 per cent of elderly people have the condition, which is usually fairly mild and can be treated simply by altering the diet, or occasionally by tablets, some of which increase the production of insulin by the pancreas. The onset is usually slow and undramatic.

In children the picture is quite different. Affecting around one child in a thousand the onset is usually sudden and treatment almost always means regular injections of insulin. Insulin cannot be taken in tablet form as it is destroyed by acids in the stomach.

Doctors have a number of different types of insulin to choose from and they will always try to choose one that gives the best control for your child's lifestyle. Parents often become expert in adjusting insulin doses if needed, by performing blood and urine tests. The more a child can learn about his diabetes the better, and some splendid books are available including one that features Rupert Bear explaining the disease for young children – in rhyme!

The more a child understands about diabetes the less resentful he will feel about any restrictions that his disease causes him. Diet is obviously important. In particular the refined carbohydrates (sweets and sugar) are best avoided. Nevertheless in recent years the advice on diabetic diet has changed radically and most diabetics are now advised to follow the same sort of diet that I recommended for everyone in Chapter 1, with more fibre, less sugar, and so on. As more families adopt this eating pattern – and all the evidence suggests that this is happening – the diabetic child will be on the same 'diet' as all the rest of us.

Children with diabetes have gone on to reach positions of eminence in almost every field of life, even including sport. It is vital to ensure your child realizes that the diagnosis is not the end of their dreams. However it may, understandably, cause immense resentment and anger at first. In time, with your help, he will take the condition for granted.

Diabetes does sometimes run in families, but this is far from inevitable. Even if both parents of a child are diabetic, there is still only a one-in-twenty chance that their child will be diabetic too. Indeed the whole cause of diabetes remains something of a mystery. One thing does seem to be certain. Children do not get diabetes by eating too many sweets, though obesity certainly makes it more common in the elderly.

It is well worth informing playgroup leaders, teachers, and your child's friends' parents about the diabetes. The less fuss that is made at mealtimes and at parties the less your child will feel unusual. However it is far better to get older children to explain the situation themselves, otherwise they will feel embarrassed and secretive! If they talk about their diabetes, they will come to terms with it far better.

Coeliac Disease

Coeliac disease is a relatively rare, but important, condition in childhood. Gluten in the diet of such children makes the fine finger-like projections of the lining of the bowel virtually disappear. The lining of the small intestine becomes smooth, and as a result is far less efficient at absorbing nutrients.

This poor absorption has two chief effects, both of which are fairly predictable. As less food is absorbed, more comes straight through and the children suffer from chronic loose motions. Secondly, the lack of nutrients getting into the body results in poor growth, poor health, and anaemia.

Gluten is found in wheat, rye, barley and oats, and the only effective treatment is to avoid gluten completely. The recovery on such a diet is usually total, but unfortunately eating gluten containing foods results in the problem flaring up again.

A gluten free diet would be relatively easy to cope with if it were not for the huge number of processed foods, soups, sauces, and so on which contain gluten. It is therefore essential for parents to get hold of detailed lists of gluten containing and gluten free foods. Dieticians will offer a great deal of help, as will the excellent Coeliac Society.

Many of the behavioural problems that children exhibit after being put on such a diet are similar to those of diabetic children. However, as Rae Ward, Consultant Dietician to the Coeliac Society, told me, the attitude of parents is all important and often coloured by the way they first learnt about the condition. As she said, 'Parents who are given plenty of time by a consultant paediatrician explaining the diagnosis and then seen at length by a good dietician have a tremendous advantage over those who leave hospital bewildered about the condition and the diet.'

It is obviously much easier if a child is diagnosed as a baby rather than in later childhood. Once a child has got used to eating Smarties, Mars Bars, ordinary bread, Wimpy's and so on he is far more likely to rebel at the prospect of a diet – even if it does make him feel better.

The extent to which children complain depends on the symptoms they get if they eat gluten. Some are violently ill, with vomiting, diarrhoea, and abdominal pain, and they are far less likely to complain than the child who has no obvious immediate effects. For such children the ban on so many types of fast food seems an unfair imposition. Holidays can be a problem too, although self-catering makes life much easier and the Coeliac Society does have details of hotels where a gluten free diet is available.

As for school meals, if you find it impossible to convey your child's needs to a school meals supervisor, send a packed lunch instead. One coeliac child I know was hardly allowed anything by a kindly but overzealous supervisor, who seemed to ban everything except meat and fruit! The child got understandably hungry.

Phenylketonuria

A very rare condition occurring in about one child in every 10,000 births, phenylketonuria (PKU) is caused by a chemical, an enzyme, being absent from the liver. This chemical normally causes the metabolism of a type of amino-acid, called phenylalanine, in the diet. If the enzyme is missing the amount of phenylalanine in the blood rises dangerously and results in brain damage and severe mental handicap.

Even though it is so rare, every child in the UK is screened for this condition as the effects can be devastating. Within a few days of birth a small blood sample is analysed, and if PKU is diagnosed a lifelong diet is required which reduces the amount of phenylalanine the child takes to safe levels.

With such a rare condition, and such an essential diet, detailed and personal dietary advice must be obtained, and an organization exists to help parents with their difficulties.

Cleft Lip and Palate

Most of the feeding problems associated with a cleft lip or palate result from an inability to suck, and therefore are far more important to babies. This difficulty in sucking results in feeds taking a long time, and food often returns down the nose.

Modern surgical repair techniques have totally changed the outlook for such children and long-term problems are very rare. The Cleft Lip and Palate Association provides much useful information and all parents of such children would be well advised to contact them.

The Handicapped

While there are a great many types of mental and physical handicap, one particular problem tends to occur with all of them – the problem of obesity.

I well remember watching a pleasant, young, but grossly obese boy with Down's syndrome stuffing himself with cakes, sweets, and sugary drinks. I mentioned this to his mother. 'I know it's wrong,' she said, 'but he has so few pleasures in life. It seems cruel to stop him.'

Is it really cruel? I can understand precisely what she meant, and I know she was being kind, but the resulting obesity, which is made worse by the relative immobility of such children, can cause immense problems. Arthritis, immobility, and all the other hazards of obesity affect the handicapped every bit as much as they affect everyone else, particularly now medical advances give such children a longer life expectancy than in the past.

Feeding problems in general are extremely common in the handicapped. It has been estimated that 80 per cent or more of severely handicapped persons have some type of feeding disorder that can lead to undesirable conse-quences for physical, social and educational development . Problems vary from obesity to food refusal, but one of the most important problems, especially with the mentally handicapped, is that they cannot be relied on to select an adequate choice of foods in the way that other children can. Given a free choice of good foods most children will end up with a more than adequate diet. The mentally handicapped child might well end up short of important nutrients, so causing them even greater problems than they already have. Parents should keep a close eye on the quality of such children's diets, and remember that many children are not able to tell them if they are hungry or thirsty.

Different handicaps obviously require specific and personal advice. Some may have difficulty chewing or swallowing. Others may not be able to sit without considerable support. Some require special feeding aids. Whatever your child's needs are, please do not struggle on alone. Your health visitor or doctor will either advise you themselves or put you in touch with groups that can. Help *is* available.

Vegetarianism

It can be very difficult to find out the truth about vegetarianism. Books and articles by vegetarians are obviously biased in one direction, while non-vegetarian writers have generally made their minds up in the other. However, I think it is possible to sum up the effects of vegetarianism on children fairly simply.

There is no evidence that vegetarian children are either more or less healthy than other children, but there is no doubt that it is harder to ensure an adequate protein intake for the vegetarian child.

Please note that I used the word 'harder' – certainly not 'impossible'. Milk, eggs, cheese, and beans can be splendid sources of protein, but a vegetarian diet needs closer supervision to ensure that a child gets all the nutrients he needs.

In particular the faddy toddler is more than likely to run into nutritional problems if he is a vegetarian. Luckily most vegetarians know far more about nutrition than most meat eaters, and can keep an eye on diet in a careful way. Vegetarianism is sometimes seen as a negative activity. They don't eat meat. To be successful it is equally important that the diet is looked at positively – in other words what they do eat is far more important than what they do not eat.

I do not want to go into the advantages and disadvantages of vegetarianism here. There are countless books on the topic already, and the world can do without another set of views. However, whilst most vegetarians are healthy, and sometimes healthier than their meat-eating friends, there is one group whose diet could be hazardous for young children.

There are three main types of vegetarian diet:

1 *Vegans, or strict vegetarians*:
   These eat no animal foods of any kind. All protein is taken from plant sources.
2 *Ovolactovegetarians*:
   These take eggs and milk, cheese, and other dairy produce, but no fish, poultry, or meat.
3 *Lactovegetarians*:
   These take milk produce such as cheese, but no eggs, meat, fish or poultry.

Of these the vegan diet is not sufficient for young children, and is inadequate during pregnancy, unless additional dietary supplements are given. There is a strong body of opinion to say that infants and very young children do need animal sources of protein if they are going to grow properly.

One study from Seattle looked at eight children aged one to five years on vegan diets, seven on ovolacto or lacto-vegetarian diets, and twelve on ordinary mixed diets. The vegan children were all described as lethargic, were of low weight, and one was seriously malnourished. Six of the seven were receiving insufficient calories to support normal growth.

Current advice has to be that it is essential that vegan children have expert dietary advice with supplements throughout childhood, and at the very least up to the age of three or four. Children who receive eggs or dairy produce can certainly have adequate nutrition and come to no disadvantage.

Finally, there is a strict form of vegetarianism known as fruitarian. This consists of fruit alone and is inadequate for health as it provides insufficient protein, fat, minerals and vitamins. Even if you yourself can manage on such a diet – and you will certainly need supplements to keep healthy – please do not subject your child to it. It is not appropriate for growing young bodies.

Conclusion

'I wish someone had told us to stop worrying when she was little. We used to get so tense and upset about Gemma's dreadful eating. We were sure it was our fault, but we couldn't think what we'd done wrong. Eventually, after we had tried everything, we just gave up, relaxed, and stopped worrying. The extraordinary thing was that when we stopped fussing, so did Gemma. It was that easy.'

While researching this book I received many letters from parents who had made the same discovery and all were keen to pass the message on. One writer ended her letter, 'I would tell parents to try not to worry about your faddy eaters. Close your ears to other people's comments. As long as your child is healthy, what is the point of worrying?'

Another mother wrote, 'I think we all change our ideas when we have children. I've now discovered that if a child won't eat then nothing will change its mind. I've learnt not to worry, and life is so much easier.'

The message from these parents, and from much of the research that I've quoted throughout the book, is that many of the expectations we have of our children before they are born are unrealistic. If the ideas you had about childrearing aren't working as you expected then don't automatically assume that you are a failure as a parent. It is far more likely that your expectations were well intentioned but misguided. There is nothing weak about treating your child as a person who has likes and dislikes, and much of the worry about children's varying appetites stems from ignorance of the natural and normal phases that all children go through.

I hope this book will have shown you that fears and worries about children's eating are tremendously common and you are certainly not alone. You will now have some guidelines on how to look at your particular problem, and how to cope with it.

By now you will have considered most of the following points:

- Is there really a problem at all, or are you comparing your child with unrealistic or unnecessary expectations?'
- Is your child growing normally – a sure sign that he must be getting reasonable nutrition?
- Are you offering portions or meals that are simply bigger than he can face?
- Are you expecting standards of mealtime behaviour – such as not reading at table – that you don't keep to yourself?
- If you are worried about your child's overall level of nutrition, have you tried keeping a detailed food diary?
- Are you making mealtimes a battle? If so, the tension will put him off his food, so making him even less likely to eat – until he asks for a between-meal snack.
- Is he having so many snacks or drinks that there is no space left for meals?
- Are you using food as a pacifier and as a bribe?
- Will your insistence that he eats up food that he

doesn't want result in a lifetime's over-eating and eventual obesity?

Eating problems are universal, but – as the parents I have quoted have discovered – they are often relatively simple to sort out. When you understand how a child grows and what a good diet should, and should not, contain then you can approach the problem in a far more logical and relaxed frame of mind.

Inevitably you will still endure times when your children worry or infuriate you. You wouldn't be a normal parent if they didn't. Nevertheless many of the worries you have had about feeding should now be in a better perspective and mealtimes will again be a pleasure.

Believe it or not, one day your son or daughter will probably get married and boast about those 'wonderful meals Mum used to make'.

Bon appétit.

Appendix

Useful Organizations

Please enclose a stamped addressed envelope when writing to these organizations. Many of them are run by volunteers on very limited funds.

British Institute of Learning
Disabilities,
Wolverhampton Rd,
Kidderminster,
Worcestershire,
DY10 3PP
    Tel : 01562 850251
    Fax : 01562 851970

Child Growth Foundation,
2 Mayfield Avenue,
London,
W4 1PW
    Tel : 0181 994 7625

CLAPA,
Cleft Lip and Palate
Association,
1, Eastwood Gardens,
Kenton,
Newcastle-upon-Tyne,
NE3 3DQ
    Tel : 0191 2859396

The Coeliac Society,
PO Box 181,
London,
NW2 2QY
    (N.B. Can only deal with medically diagnosed coeliacs)

Cystic Fibrosis Trust,
Alexandra House,
5, Blyth Road,
Bromley,
Kent,
BR1 3RS
    Tel : 0181 464 7211
    Fax : 0181 313 0472

British Diabetic Association,
10, Queen Anne Street,
London,
W1M 0BD

Eating Disorders Association,
Sackville Place,
44, Magdalen Street,
Norwich,
NR3 1JU
    Tel : 01603 621414

National Eczema Society,
163 Eversholt Street,
London,
NW1 1BU

The Hyperactive Children's
Support Group,
71, Whyke Lane,
Chichester,
West Sussex,
PO19 2LD
    Tel : 01903 725182
(Weekdays 10.00 - 15.30)

MENCAP,
(Royal Society for Mentally
Handicapped Children &
Adults)
123, Golden Lane,
London,
EC1Y 0RT
    Tel : 0171 454 0454
    Fax : 0171 608 3254

The Migraine Trust,
45 Great Ormond Street,
London,
WC1N 3HZ
    Helpline : 0171 278 2676

NSPKU,
(The National Society for
Phenylketonuria (U.K.) Ltd)
7 Southfield Close,
Willen,
Milton Keynes,
MK15 9LL
    Tel : 01908 691653

The Vegetarian Society,
Parkdale,
Dunham Rd,
Altrincham,
Cheshire,
WA14 4QG
    Tel : 0161 928 0793
    Fax : 0161 926 9182

References

Chapter 1: A Good Diet

The two major reports mentioned in this chapter were the NACNE report and the COMA report. The NACNE (National Advisory Committee on Nutrition Education) report was published by the Health Education Council in September 1983. It includes a magnificent bibliography which lists 91 important references on nutrition and health. The highly technical contents of the report were simplified for the lay reader by Dr Alan Maryon-Davis and Jane Thomas in *Diet 2000* (Pan Books, 1984)

The COMA (Committee on Medical Aspects of Food Policy) Report was published by the UK Government under the title 'Diet and Cardiovascular Disease' in July 1984.

The changes in consumption of dairy products and other foods were reported in *The Times* on 25 June 1984, and the different incidence of coronary artery disease in different societies was examined in 1970 by J. Stammler in 'Ischaemic Heart Disease' (ed. J. Hass, Leiden University Press).

The fact that lowering the level of cholesterol in the blood reduces the risk of heart disease was reported by the Lipid Research Clinic's Coronary Prevention Trial in the *Journal of the American Medical Association* in January 1984 (251:351–364 and 365–374).

Detailed charts of vitamin, protein, mineral, and other requirements are given in *Feeding Your Children* by Miranda Hall (Piatkus Books, 1984) – if you really feel you need them.

References

Chapter 2: Vitamins and Fluoride

Two very useful summaries of vitamin D deficiency have been published in recent years. The first was published by Dr William Stephens in *General Practitioner* (15 June 1984) and the second came from O. G. Brooke of St George's Hospital, London in 1983 (Arch Dis Child 58:573–4).

The case of scurvy in a twenty-four-year-old man was reported in the *BMJ* in March 1983 (286, 881).

The paper on the effect of vitamin and mineral supplementation on intelligence of a sample of schoolchildren was published in the *Lancet* in 1988 (Jan 23, pp. 140–143). A few weeks later, a large number of critical letters about this study were published in the same journal (Feb 20, pp. 407–409), and a particularly interesting exposé of the study by Caroline Richmond was reported in *General Practitioner* (Feb 26, p. 59). The 1990 study on the same topic was performed by Crombie et al and published in the *Lancet* (Mar 31 1990).

The study which suggested that a fruit-free diet carries a similar risk to the lungs as does smoking was performed by David Strachan and his colleagues and was published in 1991 in the journal *Thorax* (46: 624–629)

The significance of fluoride being swallowed by children using fluoride-containing toothpastes was raised by T. B. Dowell in 'The Use of Toothpaste in Infancy' in *British Dental Journal* (1981, 150:247–249). In the same journal in 1981 (151:118-121) Simon McDonald and his colleagues looked at the usually successful methods used by dentists for preventing caries in their own children.

An excellent review of the status of fluoride supplementation from around the world was published by O. Haugejorden and L. A. Heloe in August 1981 (Community Dent. Oral Epidemiol. 9:159-169). This showed the remarkable range of approaches that have been used, from the addition of fluoride to fruit juice to putting it into the flours used for baking bread.

Another useful review of the whole topic of fluoridation can be found in 'Fluorides in the prevention of Caries' by G. B. Winter (Arch Dis Child (1983) 58:485–487

References

Chapter 3: Normal Growth

The report on the largest baby ever born was published in the *Lancet* in 1884 by G. Eddowes (2, 941) and the effects of smoking in pregnancy on the subsequent growth of the child were reported by E. Eid in 1970 (PhD Thesis, Sheffield University). *The Times* (16 Oct 1984) reported the increasing average height of Chinese young people.

The calculations for working out a child's height as an adult are taken from Professor R. Illingworth's invaluable book *The Normal Child* (Churchill Livingstone, Edinburgh). The growth charts were published by J. M. Tanner and R. H. Whitehouse in the 'Archives of Diseases of Childhood' in 1976 (51, 170–9) where additional and more detailed charts can be consulted.

Chapter 4: Mealtimes and Manners

The research on attitudes to mealtimes by John and Elizabeth Newson was published in *Four Years Old in an Urban Community* (Pelican Books, 1970).

A review of the role of breakfast in the nutrition of five-to-twelve-year-old children was published by Karen Morgan, et al., in 1981 (Am. J. Clin. Nutr.: 34 – 1418–27).

School meals in the UK were assessed by Professor Bender and his colleagues in the *British Medical Journal* in 1972 (2, 383–385). More recent criticism of the poor nutritional value of school meals was made in a report carried out for the Inner London Education Authority and reported in *The Times* (16 Oct 1984).

The detailed analysis of food served at McDonalds Restaurants was carried out at Leatherhead Food Research Association in 1984 and published by McDonalds themselves.

The study on the nutritional status of schoolchildren in an inner city area, which showed the remarkable level of crisp and chip consumption in this age group, was published in the *Archives of Disease in Childhood* in May 1994 (pp 376–381). The report which suggested that giving iron supplements to children who did not need it could affect their growth was published in May 1994 in the *Lancet* (pp 1252–54)

Chapter 5: Food Refusal

The survey on the problems faced by parents of four-year-olds was carried out by John and Elizabeth Newson and published in *Four Years Old in an Urban Community* (Pelican Books, 1970). The American survey by Roberts and Schoelkopf entitled 'Eating, Sleeping, and Elimination Practices in a group of 2½year old children' was published in 1982 (*Am. J. Dis. Childh.* 82: 121–52).

Clara Davis, who did the research in the 1920s and 1930s on children's eating, published at least twelve papers on this topic. Perhaps one of the most important was published in the *American Journal of Diseases in Childhood* in 1928 (36: 651–79). The more recent research on the same topic was by Leann Birch and her colleagues in Illinois, and published in the *New England Journal of Medicine* in 1991 (324: 232–5).

Research that showed that parents' attempts to coerce their children into eating food they did not want is reported more often by obese adults than those of normal weight was published in the *Journal of the Society of Clinical Psychology* in 1984 (2: 305–13).

The Medical Research Council survey which showed wide variation in the diet of different children was published in 1947 but is still relevant today. The author was E. M. Widdowson, and the title was 'A Study of Individual Children's Diets' (Medical Research Council Special Report, no. 257 HMSO, 1947).

Chapter 6: Snacks and Sweets

The research on children's consumption of sweet foods and the link with such activities as television watching was reported in 'Relationships between family variables and children's prefer-ence for and consumption of sweet foods' by Nancy Ritchey and Christine Olson of Cornell University, New York (Ecology of Food & Nutrition, 1983:257–266).

Research that showed that children who see television commercials for sweet foods are more likely to choose sweet foods if given a choice of snacks was reported in 1980. (J. P. Galst in *Child Dev.* 51: 935–939). An interesting review of the effects of adult's eating on young children's acceptance of unfamiliar foods was reported by Harper and Sanders in 1975 (*J. Exp. Child. Psychol.* 20:206–214).

The comments by Graham MacGregor, director of Charing Cross Hospital's blood pressure unit, on the effect of a child's diet on his future health were reported in *The Times* (29 Oct 1984).

Chapter 7: The Underweight Child

Professor Tanner, head of the Institute of Child Health, London, gave the figures for the late referral for growth hormone deficiency at the launch of an appeal by the Child Growth Foundation, and reported in *Doctor* (13 Sept 1984).

The incidence of anorexia nervosa was discussed in a paper by A. H. Crisp, et al., in the *British Journal of Psychiatry* in 1976 (128, 549) and also by Garner and Garfinkel in the *Lancet* in 1978 (ii:674). A psychotherapeutic approach to the treatment of the condition is well discussed by H. Bruch in *The Golden Cage: the Enigma of Anorexia Nervosa* (Open Books, London, 1978). Bulimia Nervosa was discussed by G. F. Russell in 1979 (*Psychol. Med.* 9:429) in 'Bulimia Nervosa: an ominous variant of anorexia nervosa'.

Chapter 8: Obesity

The problem of the obese child was investigated at length in 1962 by M. Borjeson in *Acta Paediat. Uppsala* (51, Suppl 132) where data concerning 718 overweight girls and 687 overweight

References

boys is presented. A more recent major review was presented by W. Dietz in *The Journal of Paediatrics* (1983: 103:676–686).

The study which showed how few television actors are significantly overweight was published by Kurman in *Anorexia Nervosa : Recent Developments* in 1983 (New York: Alan R. Liss). The disturbing report on how children reacted to pictures of other children with various disabilities or problems, including obesity, was published by Goodman and colleagues in a paper entitled 'Variant reactions to physical disabilities' in the *American Sociological Review* (28 (1963) 429–435).

E. Eid showed the correlation between excessive weight gain in the first few months and obesity at six to eight years in the *British Medical Journal* (1970:ii:74) and the observation that a high proportion of obese children, as opposed to infants, became obese adults was shown by C. Peckham et al. in the same journal (286, 1237). The possible genetic origins of childhood obesity were discussed by A. G. C. Whitelaw in the *British Medical Journal* in 1976 (1, 985) and the fact that breast feeding helps prevent later obesity was shown by M. S. Kramer in *The Journal of Paediatrics* (1981:98:833).

The poor results in the long term of hospital treatment for childhood obesity were shown by O. Stark et al. in *Recent Advances in Obesity Research* in 1975 (Newman Publishing, London). J. Lloyd and O. Wolff showed in 1976 in *Recent Advances in Paediatrics* (Churchill Livingstone, London, p. 305) that obese children, can most easily be recognized by simple inspection. The important study on whether adopted children take after their natural or adoptive parents when it comes to obesity was published by Stunkard and colleagues in 'An adoption study of human obesity', in the *New England Journal of Medicine* in 1986. (314: 193–8)

The research comparing the food intake of obese and non-obese brothers was reported by Marjorie Waxman and Albert Stunkard in *The Journal of Paediatrics* in 1980 (96: 187–193). Geoffrey Cannon, in his book *Dieting Makes You Fat* (Sphere, 1984) discusses the interesting connection between dieting and changes in metabolic rate.

The study which compared the dietary input and exercise of

References

boys in the 1930s and today was based on work by Professor John Durnin of Glasgow University, and reported in *General Practitioner* (16.5.86).

Finally, a major review of the fascinating topic of brown fat and its possible effects on obesity was published in the *New England Journal of Medicine* in December 1984 (311:1549-1558) and includes an incredible list of 99 references on this topic.

Chapter 9: Sickness and Diseases

The topic of rehydration in acute diarrhoea in childhood was discussed in two papers in the *Drugs and Therapeutics Bulletin*, published by the Consumers' Association (1978:16, 1 and 1979:17, 51).

Toddler diarrhoea was reviewed by J. A. Walker-Smith in the 'Archives of Disease in Childhood' in 1980 (55, 329–30). The figures for the mortality rate in diarrhoea in infants were taken from a report by N. Barnes and N. Roberton (Update, 1979, 885–892).

The fascinating list of objects that children with pica have eaten is taken from Professor Ronald Illingworth's book *The Normal Child* (Churchill Livingstone, Edinburgh 1979). The question of anaemia in children with pica is dealt with by M. Gutelius et al. in 'Nutritional studies of children with pica' (*Pediatrics*, 1962:29, 1012).

The incidence of recurrent abdominal pain in childhood was reported by M. L. Kellmer Pringle, et al., in the *National Child Development Study* (1966, Humanities Press, London) and also in the 'Archives of Disease in Childhood' in 1958 by Apley and Naish (1958:33, 165). It was John Apley who wrote the classic medical book on this topic entitled *The Child with Abdominal Pains* (Blackwell Scientific Publications, Oxford).

The list of possible causes of recurrent pains was reported by J. A. Dodge in the *British Medical Journal* (1976, 1, 385–7). The long-term prognosis for such children was discussed by M. Christensen and O. Mortensen in 1978 (*Archives of Disease in Childhood*, 50: 110–14). The question of whether recurrent abdominal pain is a psychogenic disorder was raised by McGrath et al. in 1983 (*Arch Dis Childh*, 1983:58:888–890).

Chapter 10: Allergies and Additives

An excellent brief review of current views on food allergy is given in a leading article in *The New England Journal of Medicine* in August 1984 (Vol 311, 399–400) and the April 1984 issue of *The Journal of the Royal College of Physicians* gave a more detailed overview of this important topic (1984:18:83-123).

The report on the risks of strict diets was produced by researchers from Manchester and reported in the *Archives of Disease in Childhood* (1984, 59, 323).

A simple guide to E Numbers called *Look at the Label* can be obtained free from the Ministry of Agriculture, Fisheries, and Food, whilst a more detailed guide can be found in *E for Additives* by Maurice Hanssen and Jill Marsden (Thorsons, 1984).

Among the many papers that have reviewed the place of food additives in behavioural problems, the research by Swanson and Kinsbourne in *Science* (207:1485) is one of the most interesting, and concluded that additives did affect performance at learning tests. Taking an opposite viewpoint, Eric Taylor of the Institute of Psychiatry in London reviewed three recent reviews of this topic in the *Archives of Disease in Childhood* (1984, 59, 97–8) and concluded that any helpful results were largely due to a placebo effect. In contrast, the important and positive 1993 study on the effects of a 'few food diet' in hyperactive children was published by Carter, and colleagues from the Institute of Child Health in London, in the *Archives of Disease in Childhood*. (69: 564–568).

Chapter 11: Special Problems and Special Diets

The various self-help groups produce publications which are tremendously useful, but are not listed here. The appendix gives the addresses of the various organizations. However a good overall view of the topic is given in *Diets for Sick Children* by D. Francis (Blackwell, Oxford, 1980).

A magnificent bibliography listing 96 separate references on eating problems in the mentally handicapped can be found on pages 22–26 of a book entitled *Life Training Behaviour – Analysis and Intervention* edited by Meyer and Hollis and published by the American Association of Mental Deficiency in 1982. An interesting treatment approach is detailed in *Behavioural Treatment of Food Refusal and Selectivity in Developmentally Disabled Children* by Mary Riordan and her colleagues from the Johns Hopkins University School of Medicine and the John F. Kennedy Institute in *Applied Research in Mental Retardation*, Vol 1, 95–112 (1980). The estimates of the incidence of feeding problems in the handicapped comes from R. Perske, et al., in *Mealtimes for severely and profoundly handicapped persons: New concepts and attitudes* published by the University Park Press of Baltimore in 1977.

An assessment of the risks faced by children receiving certain strict diets was reported in the *British Medical Journal* in 1979 (Malnutrition in infants receiving cult diets: a form of child abuse – *B.M.J.*, 1979, i, 296–298). A review entitled 'Bizarre and unusual diets' was published in the *Practitioner* in 1979 (222:643–647) and this looked at such diets as the fruitarian and zen macrobiotic diets.

INDEX

Index

Index